P.G. BARTON

Vitamin Deficiency in the Elderly

Prevalence, Clinical Significance
and Effects on Brain Function

Vitamin Deficiency in the Elderly

Prevalence, Clinical Significance
and Effects on Brain Function

EDITED BY

J.R. Kemm

MD, MRCP, MFCM
Senior Lecturer in Social Medicine
Department of Social Medicine
University of Birmingham

WITH THE ASSISTANCE OF

R.J. Ancill

MA, MB, BChir, MRCPsych
Clinical Associate Professor of Psychiatry
University of British Columbia
Vancouver

Blackwell Scientific Publications
OXFORD LONDON EDINBURGH
BOSTON PALO ALTO MELBOURNE

© 1985 by
Blackwell Scientific Publications
Editorial offices:
Osney Mead, Oxford, OX2 0EL
8 John Street, London, WC1N
2ES
23 Ainslie Place, Edinburgh,
EH3 6AJ
52 Beacon Street, Boston
Massachusetts 02108, USA
667 Lytton Avenue, Palo Alto
California 94301, USA
107 Barry Street, Carlton
Victoria 3053, Australia

First published 1985

Set by Colset Pte Ltd, Singapore
Printed and bound by
Billing and Sons Ltd, Worcester

DISTRIBUTORS

USA
  Blackwell Mosby Book
    Distributors
  11830 Westline Industrial
    Drive
  St Louis, Missouri 63141

Canada
  Blackwell Mosby Book
    Distributors
  120 Melford Drive,
    Scarborough
  Ontario M1B 2X4

Australia
  Blackwell Scientific
    Publications (Australia)
    Pty Ltd
  107 Barry Street, Carlton
  Victoria 3053

British Library
Cataloguing in Publication Data

Vitamin deficiency in the elderly:
prevalence, clinical significance
and effects on brain function.
    1. Aged——Diseases
    2. Deficiency diseases
    3. Vitamins in human nutrition
    I. Kemm, J.R.   II. Ancill, R.J.
    618.97'639   RC962.5

ISBN 0-632-01365-6

Contents

List of Contributors

R.J. Ancill

MA, MB, BChir, MRCPsych
Clinical Associate Professor of Psychiatry, University of British
Columbia, Vancouver, Canada

M.H. Briscoe

MRCPsych
University of Wales College of Medicine, Whitchurch Hospital,
Cardiff, CF4 7XB

M.L. Burr

MD, MFCM
Epidemiologist, M.R.C. Epidemiology Unit (South Wales), 4 Richmond Road, Cardiff, CF2 3AS

A.C. Carr

MA, AKC, MB, BS, MRCS, MRCP, MRCPsych, MPhil
Department of Psychopharmacology, Institute of Psychiatry,
London, SE5 8AF

K.O. Chung-a-on

BSc
Department of Biochemistry, University of Surrey, Guildford,
Surrey GU2 5XH

J.W.T. Dickerson

PhD, FIBiol
Professor of Human Nutrition, Division of Nutrition and Food
Science, Department of Biochemistry, University of Surrey,
Guildford, Surrey, GU2 5XH

J. Greenwood
BSc, PhD
Research Assistant, Institute of Psychiatry, London, SE5 8AF

J.R. Kemm
MD, MRCP, MFCM
Senior Lecturer in Social Medicine, Department of Social Medicine, University of Birmingham, Birmingham, B15 2TJ

W.H. MacLennan
MD, FRCP
Reader in Geriatric Medicine, Department of Medicine, Ninewells Hospital & Medical School, Dundee, DD1 9SY

O.E. Pratt
DSc, FRCPath
Reader in Experimental Chemical Pathology, Institute of Psychiatry, London, SE5 8AF

J.H. Puxty
MB, ChB, MRCP
Lecturer in Medicine, Department of Geriatric Medicine, Hope Hospital, Eccles Old Road, Pendleton, Salford, Lancashire, M5 2AA

D.M. Shaw
FRCP, PhD, FRCPsych
Consultant Psychiatrist, Biochemical Psychiatry Laboratory, Department of Psychological Medicine, Whitchurch Hospital, Welsh National School of Medicine, Cardiff, CF4 7XB

G.K. Shaw
FRCPsych, DPM
Consultant Psychiatrist, Bexley Hospital, Bexley, Kent, DA5 2BW

D.E. Thomas

SRD
Senior I Dietician, St James' Hospital, Locksway Road, Portsmouth, PO4 8LD

A.D. Thomson

PhD, FRCP(Ed)
Consultant Physician, Greenwich District Hospital, London, SE10. Honary Senior Lecturer, Kings College Hospital, Denmark Hill, London, SE5 8RX

D.I. Thurnham

BSc, PhD
Top Grade Biochemist, Head of Nutrition Section, Clinical Investigation Unit, Dudley Road Hospital, Birmingham, B18 7QH

S.F. Tidmarsh

BSc
University of Wales College of Medicine, Whitchurch Hospital, Cardiff, CF4 7XB

Preface

There is a widespread feeling that a significant amount of ill-health in the elderly is caused by poor nutrition and, in particular, by deficiency of micronutrients. It is obviously important to establish to what extent this is true since nutritional deficiency is eminently preventable and treatable. Unfortunately the evidence linking nutrition and health in old age is fragmentary and difficult to interpret.

A symposium on 'Vitamin Deficiency in the Elderly' was held at the Postgraduate Centre, Queen Elizabeth Hospital, Birmingham in June 1984. This book is a more detailed review of the same topic and sets out to explore the questions as to how common vitamin deficiency is in the elderly, how clinical signs and biochemical indicators of nutritional status are to be interpreted, and what evidence there is that vitamin deficiency when present, causes ill-health in the elderly.

The production of this book has been made possible by the generous support of Bencard. I also thank my secretary Mrs P. Wills whose good humour and skill have helped so much in the production of this book. Finally I thank Cathy, Emma and Jeremy who did not complain when I spent too much time working on the manuscript and too little time with them.

John Kemm

1 The Concept of Vitamin Deficiency

J.R. Kemm

' 'When I use a word', Humpty Dumpty said in rather
a scornful tone, 'it means just what I choose it to mean
— neither more, nor less'.'

Through the Looking Glass, Lewis Carroll

Words and phrases tend to change their meanings and different
authors all too often use the same words with different meanings. This book is about vitamin deficiency in the elderly, but it is
important to be precise as to what those words mean.

Textbooks of medicine describe a group of diseases classified
as vitamin deficiency states. These diseases have four cardinal
features:

1   they have characteristic symptoms and signs
2   they are caused by a dietary deficiency of a specific vitamin
3   they are cured by administration of very small amounts of
that specific vitamin
4   there are specific biochemical abnormalities.

The concept of vitamin deficiency embodied in these textbook
descriptions is easily understood and is based on the disease
patterns seen in children and young adults. The understanding
of the vitamin deficiency states which are usually described in
the elderly requires a rather different concept.

THE VITAMIN CONCEPT

A short historical review is helpful in understanding how the
textbook concept of vitamin deficiency developed, and how that
concept has subsequently been expanded.

A vitamin is an organic substance which is necessary in very
small amounts for normal growth and health. This idea is so
familiar to us that it is difficult to realise how revolutionary it
was when first postulated. In the late 19th century various diseases such as scurvy, beriberi, rickets and xerophthalmia were
suspected to be caused by inadequate food but there was no

1

clear understanding of the nature of the deficiency. Carbo-
hydrates, fats, proteins and certain minerals had been
recognised as components of the diet and were generally
believed to be all that was needed.

Casimir Funk was one of the first to suggest that in addition to
these substances very small amounts of other nutrients were
required. He suggested that lack of these nutrients might be the
cause of dietary deficiency diseases (Funk 1912) and coined the
term 'vital amines' or 'vitamines' to describe them.

Gowland Hopkins working in Cambridge provided further
evidence for this proposition by showing in carefully controlled
experiments that rats fed a diet adequate in fat, protein, carbohydrate and minerals failed to thrive unless they were also given
small volumes of milk. He argued that the milk contained insignif-
icant amounts of known nutrients and must therefore contain
some 'accessory factor' absent from the basic diet but necessary
in very small quantities for normal growth (Hopkins 1912).

Later workers isolated and elucidated the structure of the
various vitamins and showed that Hopkin's 'accessory factors'
and Funk's vitamines' were the same. The name was changed to
vitamin when it was realised that most were not amines. Various
animal models of deficiency disease were developed and shown
to respond to addition of specific vitamins to the diet while deficiency diseases in man were also found to respond to specific
vitamin therapy. Developments in biochemistry showed that
most vitamins functioned as co-enzymes which explained how
nutrients in such small quantities could have such profound
effects.

Although there are problems with our definition of vitamins
(see Chapter 6) the concept of vitamins has provided a basis for
understanding a wide variety of nutritional deficiency diseases.

VITAMIN DEFICIENCY IN THE ELDERLY

The role of vitamins in prevention of classical deficiency disease
was well established in the first part of this century. With the
improved standard of living and more equitable distribution
of food there was a feeling that nutritional deficiency had
been virtually eradicated in the United Kingdom (Drummond &

Wilbraham 1958; DHSS 1978). This euphoric picture was disturbed by a series of reports suggesting that in the elderly and some other groups nutritional deficiency was still common.

Clinical signs supposedly indicative of nutritional deficiency such as follicular keratosis, petechial and sheet haemorrhages, cheilosis, angular stomatitis, dyssebacea and glossitis were reported to be common in elderly patients in hospital (Taylor 1968) and in the elderly at home (Taylor *et al.* 1971).

Dietary surveys revealed that the elderly often had low intakes of vitamins (Exton-Smith & Stanton 1965; DHSS 1972; MacLeod *et al.* 1974; Lonergan *et al.* 1975; DHSS 1979a; Vir & Love 1979).

Blood levels of vitamin C were commonly low in hospitalised (Batata *et al.* 1967; Griffiths *et al.* 1967; Wilson *et al.* 1972; Schorah *et al.* 1979; Vir & Love 1979; Kemm & Allcock 1984) and non-hospitalised elderly (Milne *et al.* 1971; Burr *et al.* 1974a; DHSS 1979a). Raised levels of transketolase activation coefficient suggestive of thiamin deficiency (Griffiths *et al.* 1967; DHSS 1979a; Vir & Love 1979; Kemm & Allcock 1984) and raised levels of erythrocyte glutathione reductase activation coefficient suggestive of riboflavin deficiency (DHSS 1979a; Vir & Love 1979; Kemm & Allcock 1984) are frequently found in the elderly. Plasma or RBC folate levels are often found to be low (Hurdle & Picton-Williams 1966; Batata *et al.* 1967; Girdwood, Thomson & Williamson 1967; DHSS 1972; 1979a; Vir & Love 1979). Histological features suggestive of osteomalacia (Aaron *et al.* 1974; Campbell *et al.* 1984) and low serum levels of 25-hydroxycholecalciferol (Corless *et al.* 1975; Nayal *et al.* 1978; MacLennan *et al.* 1979) are also common in the elderly.

There is no dispute that minor abnormalities of the types listed in the preceding paragraphs are common in the elderly, but the interpretation of these findings (further explored in Chapter 2 (intake), Chapter 3 (clinical signs) and Chapter 4 (biochemistry)) is highly contentious.

THE EXTENDED CONCEPT OF VITAMIN DEFICIENCY

Much confusion has been caused by the failure to distinguish between the dramatic clinical pictures described in classical deficiency states and the features usually considered indicative of vitamin deficiency in the elderly today. Two features of the classical concept of vitamin deficiency, the characteristic and specific symptoms and signs and the dramatic response to vitamin therapy are usually absent from modern reports of vitamin deficiency in the elderly.

The concept of vitamin deficiency has been stretched to include isolated findings of low vitamin intakes or single clinical signs or biochemical abnormalities in the absence of overt classical vitamin deficiency states. These conditions may or may not represent very early stages in the development of classical deficiency but their severity is clearly of a different order of magnitude.

HOST AND ENVIRONMENTAL FACTORS IN VITAMIN DEFICIENCY

A more critical examination suggests that the textbook concept of vitamin deficiency was always an abstraction. The historical outbreaks of deficiency disease occurred in populations ravaged by infectious diseases and subsisting on diets which were deficient in many vitamins. Lind (1753) describes 'flux' or diarrhoea as a characteristic feature of scurvy but modern accounts do not include this symptom which may well have been due to coincident infection. There are many reports (see Chapter 7) of vitamin deficiency states precipitated by infectious disease. It is clear that in many cases low dietary intake of vitamins is not a sufficient cause of vitamin deficiency states. The clinical picture of vitamin deficiency is determined not simply by the vitamin intake but also by numerous host and environmental factors.

Primary and Secondary deficiency

The role of other factors is recognised by dividing vitamin deficiency states into:

1   *primary*, where the vitamin requirement is normal and the vitamin intake is insufficient to supply that normal requirement

2   *secondary*, where the vitamin requirement is increased and the vitamin intake is insufficient to meet that increased requirement.

Pernicious anaemia is a familiar example of a secondary vitamin deficiency. The intake of vitamin B_{12} in patients with this disease is no less than that of the general population. The requirement for B_{12}, however, is greatly increased due to lack of intrinsic factor and a failure to absorb the vitamin. Pellagra in those treated with isoniazid is another familiar example of a secondary vitamin deficiency state. There is probably an element of increased requirement in the pathogenesis of all vitamin deficiency. There can be no absolute distinction between primary and secondary vitamin deficiency, but at a practical level the distinction is useful.

In view of the physiological changes of ageing and the multiple pathologies which so often accompany it, much of what is described as vitamin deficiency in the elderly may be secondary rather than primary. For the same reasons we may expect that the manifestations of vitamin deficiency in the elderly will be different and less specific than the classical deficiency states.

REVERSIBILITY OF DEFICIENCY STATES

Response to treatment with a specific vitamin is usually accepted as a criterion of classical vitamin deficiency states but some advanced deficiency states are accepted as irreversible. The disorganised eye of keratomalacia (vitamin A deficiency) and the degenerated nerve tracts of subacute combined degeneration (B_{12} deficiency) are not restored by specific therapy. Failure of specific vitamin therapy to reverse pathology in the elderly does not necessarily rule out vitamin deficiency as a contributory factor to the development of that pathology.

THE ICEBERG OF DEFICIENCY

'. . . There is a small number of individuals who are obviously malnourished . . . but apart from this limited problem there is a further more common group in which doubt arises as to whether a state of subclinical malnutrition may exist.' (DHSS 1970).

One interpretation of isolated low vitamin intakes or clinical signs or abnormal biochemistry in the elderly is that they represent subclinical malnutrition. Epidemiologists talk of the iceberg of disease by which they mean that just as the visible part of an iceberg above the water represents only one seventh of its total mass so overt disease (in this case classical vitamin deficiency) represents only a small fraction of the total pathology in the population. Subclinical vitamin deficiency which is far more common than overt deficiency is the hidden bulk of the problem (Figure 1.1). This concept of the iceberg of vitamin deficiency is beguiling but needs critical scrutiny. Are biochemical abnormalities in the elderly really associated with any morbidity and do they really represent a step toward overt deficiency? We know that the vast majority of patients with biochemical abnormalities do not progress to classical deficiency states since the former are extremely common while the latter are rare. The main evidence for the iceberg model and for this progression comes from experimentally induced deficiency in man and animals.

ANIMAL MODELS OF DEFICIENCY

It should be relatively easy to demonstrate progression through the various levels of vitamin deficiency in animals, however, most studies have concentrated on severe deficiency and little attention has been paid to the intermediate stages.

Hughes *et al.* (1980) showed that in guinea pigs on a vitamin C deficient diet, reduced tissue levels and disturbed carnitine metabolism preceded the development of overt deficiency. Rats developing riboflavin deficiency show a sequence of changes with erythrocyte glutathione reductase activation coefficients

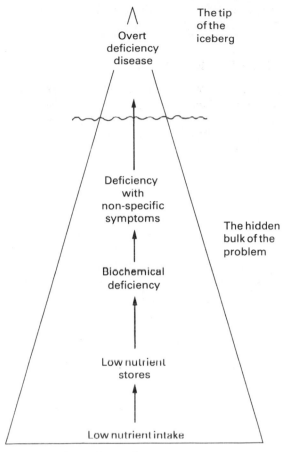

Fig. 1.1   The Iceberg of Nutritional Deficiency.

rising early while changes in other enzymes and probably more severe pathology occurred later (Prentice & Bates 1981). These animal models show that the iceberg model is applicable to some situations but their relevance to vitamin deficiency in elderly humans is debatable.

EXPERIMENTAL DEFICIENCY IN MAN

Longitudinal studies of the development of vitamin deficiency in man could show whether non specific ill-health preceded the appearance of overt deficiency and give the best evidence for the iceberg model. However such experiments are technically very difficult, cannot be continued for very long periods and for ethical reasons must be halted before severe deficiency develops.

There have been several studies of experimental vitamin C deficiency in man. A group of volunteers in Sheffield was fed a diet very low in vitamin C. Although they developed follicular keratitis, gingivitis and other clinical signs of early scurvy after about 20 weeks, they did not complain of general pains, weakness or of non specific ill-health (Krebs 1953). The study was repeated in the USA using convict volunteers and a vitamin C free diet. Similar clinical findings were made in this study but depression, anxiety and hypochondriasis were reported to develop before the clinical signs (Kinsman & Hood 1971).

In experimental thiamin deficiency general malaise and irritability were reported to occur after biochemical changes and before the onset of early signs of clinical beriberi (Brin 1964). Mild personality changes were detected by sensitive psychological testing in volunteers made severely deficient in riboflavin.

The difficulties of vitamin depletion studies in man have been graphically described (Hodges *et al.* 1969). Their study began with 6 'volunteers' from the Iowa State penitentiary, but 'two escaped on the 54th day of deficiency' and 'one developed a severe anxiety reaction following his testimony concerning the escape of his companions'. The vitamin C free liquid formula diet used 'becomes monotonous and intolerable if the subjects are required to drink it' but 'they soon learn to swallow a nasogastric tube without discomfort and to administer the formula through this tube'. Being the subject of a vitamin depletion experiment is not a pleasant experience and inevitably involves consuming very dull food and accepting other irksome restrictions. This makes it extremely difficult to determine whether any minor symptoms, such as depression, anxiety and irritability which the subject may experience are due to vitamin deficiency, or the rather trying conditions of the experiment.

It has been possible to perform experimental deficiency studies under artificial conditions on younger adults but not in the elderly. The results of such studies, however, lend some support to the idea that vitamin deficiency causes non-specific ill health before the development of overt deficiency disease.

CONCLUSION

Most reports of vitamin deficiency in the elderly in the UK are radically different from the classical deficiency diseases described in textbooks. The term vitamin deficiency has been extended so that it covers not only overt deficiency disease but also low vitamin intakes, abnormal biochemistry and isolated clinical signs in the absence of overt deficiency disease. There is no doubt that such findings are common in the elderly but doubt remains whether they really indicate subclinical malnutrition and whether they are causally associated with increased morbidity. These questions are explored in subsequent chapters.

2 Recommended Intakes and Dietary Assessment

J.R. Kemm

This chapter is concerned with two deceptively simple questions. How much of each vitamin does an elderly person require and how much of each vitamin is he or she consuming?

RECOMMENDED DAILY AMOUNTS

Table 2.1 is taken from 'Recommended daily intakes of food, energy and nutrients for groups of people in the United Kingdom' (DHSS 1979b) and shows the values for elderly people. Similar tables, many of which are listed by Truswell (1976) have been produced for use in other countries. The first half of this chapter will explain why these tables must be used with caution. Their limitations are well explained in the following quotation from the preamble to the UK tables.

'It is not possible to estimate the probability that an individual is malnourished by comparing his or her intake with the recommended amount. Nevertheless it would be true to say that on present knowledge the greater the proportion of people with intakes below those recommended, the greater the possibility that some individuals may be undernourished with respect to the nutrient or nutrients in question' (DHSS 1979b).

The recommended daily amounts (RDA) 'represents a judgement of the average requirement plus a margin of safety' (DHSS 1979b). The data on which the estimate of average requirements is based are fragmentary and are usually derived from studies on young adults. The 'margin of safety' added to the average requirement would ideally be based on a knowledge of the distribution of requirements within the population, however in practice this has to be decided in the absence of such knowledge.

The RDA of vitamins for the elderly is the same (or in the case of thiamin the same relative to energy) as that for young adults.

Table 2.1   Recommended daily intakes of enmergy and nutrients for groups of elderly people in the UK (from DHSS 1979).

	Men		Women	
	65–74	75 +	55–74	75 +
Energy (cal)	2400	2150	1900	1680
(MJ)	10.0	9.0	8.0	7.0
Protein (g)	60	54	47	42
Calcium (mg)	500	500	500	500
Iron (mg)	10	10	10	10
Thiamin (mg)	1.0	0.9	0.8	0.7
Riboflavin (mg)	1.6	1.6	1.3	1.3
Nicotinic acid (mg)	18	18	15	15
Ascorbic acid (mg)	30	30	30	30
Vitamin A (μg retinol equiv.)	750	750	750	750
Vitamin D* (μg cholecalciferol)	2.5	2.5	2.5	2.5

* If exposure to sunlight is inadequate
A recommendation of 300 μg for total folate was included in the first printing but excluded from subsequent reprints.

However, since the vitamin requirement of the elderly has been estimated by uncertain extrapolation from very crude estimates of the requirements of young adults, the correctness of these RDA of vitamins for the elderly is debatable.

Such data as there are on vitamin requirements suggests that individuals vary considerably and unless the 'margin of safety' is very wide the RDA will be less than the requirement of some individuals in the population.

Optimum or minimum intake

The RDA of vitamins is derived from an estimate of average requirement which may be based on:
1   the minimum intake which is associated with the absence of any signs of deficiency disease within the community
2   the minimum intake needed to cure signs of deficiency
3   the minimum intake needed to maintain tissue saturation.
The minimum vitamin intake needed to maintain tissue saturation is much higher than the minimum intake needed to prevent or cure deficiency disease; for example, 10 mg/day are needed to prevent scurvy (Bartley, et al. 1953) but about 100 mg/day are needed for saturation (Kallner et al. 1979). Other vitamins such as A, D and B_{12} accumulate in the body but it is uncertain whether such accumulation is always beneficial (McLaren 1980).

Many have argued that RDAs should be based not on minimum requirements but on requirements for optimum health. While superficially attractive, the concept of optimum requirements raises formidable difficulties. In animal nutrition growth rate, reproductive performance, longevity, disease resistance and serum or tissue nutrient levels have all been used as criteria for assessing nutrient requirement. However, the nutrient intake to optimise these different indices of health are frequently incompatible. In rats, high nutrient intakes which maximise growth rate and reproductive performance are associated with reduced life expectancy (Munro 1981) and increased tumour incidence (Roe 1981).

In elderly humans, longevity, freedom from disease and the quality of life would be appropriate criteria for optimal health. The relationships between these indices and nutrient intake is virtually unknown though there is some evidence to suggest that a high intake of energy (and therefore of other nutrients) is associated with increased survival and above average health (Stanton & Exton-Smith 1970; DHSS 1979a). With the present state of knowledge, minimum requirements are the only practical basis for RDAs of vitamins.

International comparisons

RDAs of vitamins have varied over time and show geographical variation. The US National Research Council has repeatedly changed its RDA of vitamin C for adult men from 75 mg in 1942, to 70 mg in 1964, to 60 mg in 1968, to 45 mg in 1974, and to 60 mg in 1980. The RDA of vitamin C for adult men is 30 mg/day in the UK, Canada, Finland and Malaya, 50 mg/day in Colombia, Finland and Netherlands, 55 mg/day in South America, 60 mg/day in Indonesia, USA and Japan, 70 mg/day in East Germany, 75 mg/day in West Germany and 70–100 mg/day in USSR (Truswell 1976). A small part of this variation may be accounted for by differences in the populations for which they were designed but the size of the variation reflects the uncertainty over RDA.

Individual variation

Females are believed to have lower requirements of energy and some B vitamins than males and the requirements change with age. Some allowance for age and sex is made in the RDAs though the age-bands used are wide. Nutrient requirement is affected by activity. RDAs for the elderly usually assume a sedentary lifestyle and due allowance must be made for increased activity when present. Body size is another factor which affects nutrient requirements and some adjustment must be made in the requirement of those whose body size is very different from the average, for their age sex group.

The environment also affects an individual's nutrient requirement. Dietary requirement of vitamin D depends on sun exposure. Those with plentiful sun exposure may not need vitamin D in the diet. Low environmental temperatures increase requirement for energy and probably for vitamin A (Rodriguez & Irwin 1972).

Even when allowance has been made for age, sex, activity and environment, large differences remain in the nutrient requirements of individuals. Adult requirement for vitamin A was found to range from 525–1200 μg/day (Rodriguez & Irwin 1972) and that for vitamin B_{12} from 0.5–2.5 μg/day (Herbert

1968). Vitamin requirements depend on absorption, metabolism, distribution through the tissue and excretion. Absorption of vitamin C (Lim *et al.* 1984) and vitamin D (Barragry *et al.* 1978) may be reduced in the elderly, but that of B_{12} (McEvoy *et al.* 1982) and thiamin (Thomson 1966) is probably not affected by ageing. 25-Hydroxylation of vitamin D is reduced in the elderly (Rushton 1978). In general the effect of ageing on vitamin handling and requirement is poorly understood.

Pathological variation

RDA refers to healthy individuals and 'do not cover any additional needs arising from disease such as infections, disorders of the gastrointestinal tract or metabolic abnormalities' (DHSS 1979). However, very many of the elderly have some pathology or take some medication which may increase nutrient requirement.

Malabsorption may increase the requirement for several vitamins especially A, D and folate. Thyrotoxicosis increases the requirement for energy and some B vitamins. Renal disease may affect the metabolism of vitamin D and even minor increases in plasma creatinine are associated with increased osteoid suggesting an increased requirement for vitamin D (Kemm *et al.* 1984). The distribution of vitamin C throughout the body compartments is affected by many illnesses including infection (MacLennan & Hamilton 1977a), myocardial infarction (Vallance *et al.* 1978) and surgery (Irvin *et al.* 1978).

It is prudent to conclude that many elderly persons have vitamin requirements increased by disease processes. Increased vitamin requirements due to drug therapy are probably equally common (see Chapter 11).

Body Stores, Adaptation and Requirements

When a well-nourished animal is subjected to nutritional stress such as inadequate supply of one or more nutrients that animal will react in such a way as to minimise, or undo entirely, the effects of the nutritional stress (Mitchell 1964). This nutritional adaptation is brought about by changes in absorption, excretion, metabolism and utilisation of nutrients and will allow man to live for long periods on vitamin intakes below his long-term requirement. The vitamin requirement of an individual may be profoundly affected by his state of adaptation.

Body stores of some vitamins such as vitamins B_{12}, A and D are large relative to daily requirements, while those of vitamin C and folate are smaller. Depletion of these body stores is an important adaptive mechanism. Depletion experiments such as those with vitamin A (Rodriguez & Irwin 1972), folate (Herbert 1968) and vitamin C (Hodges *et al.* 1971) illustrate the importance of the stores in delaying the development of functional impairment. It is debatable at what point depletion of body stores ceases to be a normal adaptive mechanism and becomes a pathological change.

25-Hydroxylation of vitamin D by the liver and 1-hydroxylation by the kidney is regulated by vitamin D intake and constitutes a protective mechanism against both vitamin D deficiency and intoxication. Vitamin C might be synthesised endogenously during C depletion (Rajalakshmi *et al.* 1965). Absorption of several vitamins such as vitamin C (Mayersohn 1972) is more complete when vitamin intake is low. Conversion of β carotene to retinol is greatest when vitamin A status is low.

Adaptation to low vitamin intakes is poorly understood and its importance in the elderly even less so. In general ageing is characterised by reduced adaptive capacity, but it is not clear to what extent this includes adaptation to low vitamin intakes. Body stores of some vitamins such as vitamin A (Huque 1982) are reduced with ageing. The elderly enter old age with an accumulation of nutritional past history and the nutritional scars of youth may well affect their nutritional requirements in later life. Many of the elderly today have experienced food shortage during the years of the depression and the Second World War.

Nutrient interactions

Vitamins are eaten not as pure substances but as components of complex mixtures in food. The vitamin requirement will vary depending on the food mixture in which the vitamin is eaten.

The interaction of carbohydrate intake and thiamin was one of the first to be recognised. Beriberi was infrequent during famine but appeared when food supplies improved. Thiamin pyrophosphate is a cofactor for an enzyme in the glycolytic pathway (pyruvate decarboxylase) and the greater the energy intake the greater the thiamin requirement. Those with a high intake of alcohol also have an increased thiamin requirement. This energy dependence may be allowed for by stating the thiamin requirement relative to energy intake (mg/MJ), rather than in absolute terms.

Fibre intakes of Western countries are low and most nutritionists suggest that they should be increased, however this would then modify the requirement for several vitamins. Absorption of vitamins B_{12}, B_6 and C (Keltz, et al. 1978) may be modified by dietary fibre. Many types of fibre are rich in phytate which may impair calcium absorption and increase requirement for vitamin D.

Some vitamins can be made from precursors. The amino acid tryptophan can, for example, be converted to nicotinic acid. The requirement for this vitamin is accordingly reduced when the dietary supply of tryptophan is plentiful. Similarly β carotene can be hydrolysed in the body to produce vitamin A. The pro vitamins are allowed for in food tables by equating 60 mg tryptophan to 1 mg of nicotinic acid and 6 μg of β carotene to 1 μg of vitamin A, and then quoting values for 'nicotinic acid equivalents' and 'retinol equivalents'. Such calculations however can only be crude approximations and individuals will vary considerably as to the efficiency with which they make the conversions.

The nature of the protein in the diet may affect the distribution of vitamin C (Williams & Hughes 1972) and diets rich in leucine may increase the requirement for nicotinic acid (Gopalan 1969). The requirement for vitamin E is reduced when selenium intake is high (Levander 1975) and increased where the diet is rich in polyunsaturates. Large doses of vitamin E increase the requirement for vitamin A (Klaui 1979).

Folate metabolism is modified when the diet is deficient in vitamin C (Stokes et al. 1975) though this interaction was not apparent in the elderly (Bates et al. 1980). The complex interaction between folate and vitamin B_{12} has long been recognised and tissue levels of most B vitamins are affected by dosing with almost any other B vitamin (Dastur et al. 1976).

There are a vast number of possible nutrient interactions but fortunately in individuals eating a varied diet which provides far more than their minimum requirements these interactions are quantitatively unimportant. However, in elderly persons eating diets in which the supply of vitamins is marginal nutrient interactions may make the difference between just sufficient and not quite enough. Nutrient interactions may also be important when pharmacological doses of vitamins are given.

Conclusions

The foregoing discussion in this chapter demonstrates that a complex web of interacting factors determine the vitamin requirement of each individual. Recommended Daily Amounts (RDAs) are a useful crude guide but no substitute for skilled judgement in assessing the adequacy of nutrient intake in each individual elderly person.

MEASURING NUTRIENT INTAKE

The rest of this chapter is concerned with the question of how the vitamin intake of the elderly can be measured. No method is entirely satisfactory and any measurement must be a compromise between accuracy and completeness of assessment on the one hand and ease, speed and cheapness on the other.

The purpose of an investigation must be decided before the most appropriate method can be selected. Assessment of nutrient intake may be undertaken to investigate either the nutritional status of an individual or else the nutritional status of a group. The intention may be either to assess the absolute nutrient intake or merely to rank in order of magnitude of nutrient intakes. The particular vitamin whose intake is being studied and the ability of the subjects to cooperate with the measurement will also influence the choice of method.

Some elderly may be physically frail or confused and unable to cooperate with more complex methods. It may be better to choose a less accurate method which can be used to assess most subjects rather than a more accurate method which can only be applied to the fittest few.

Measurement of Current Intake

Most methods attempt to measure the intake over a defined short period of time. Duplicate meal analysis involves preparation of one meal for consumption and another for analysis together with recovery and analysis of plate waste. This method is precise but is extremely expensive and requires a great deal of subject cooperation. It is also probable that intake under these conditions of measurement will differ considerably from intake at other times. The only place of duplicate meal analysis is in short-term studies of the relation between nutrient intake and physiological variables in small numbers of subjects.

A slightly less arduous assessment of intake may be obtained by use of weighed dietary records. The subjects record and weigh all foods prior to consumption so that an accurate record of weights of food eaten, is obtained. Food tables are used to convert food intakes to nutrient intakes. Considerable subject cooperation and expert dietitian time are necessary for this method. It is also subject to the objection that the process of weighing and recording may temporarily disturb the subject's intake.

A further simplification is to record food consumption in terms of household measures such as teaspoons, cupfulls, medium sized potatoes, and so on. These measures can then be converted into weights from which nutrient intakes can be calculated. This method though simpler than weighing still requires considerable and sustained subject cooperation.

An alternative to prospective methods is diet recall in which the subject is asked to recall all food eaten over a period in the recent past (usually 24 hours). Estimation of quantities is a particular problem in recall methods. Recall methods are highly dependent on the skill of the interviewer. The method depends on the ability of the subject to remember what they have eaten and cannot be used with confused elderly people.

Improving intake estimates

Each of these methods offers considerable potential for error to creep in. Maintaining the subject's enthusiasm and cooperation is crucial and frequent visits from the investigator are necessary to maintain record quality. Data collection from a confused subject may require the investigator to be present at the preparation of every meal and good quality records are more easily obtained from the elderly living in residential institutions than from the elderly at home. Frequent checking of records with the subject by a skilled dietitian will permit early detection and correction of errors. Monitoring larder stores and shopping baskets can provide an independent check and reveal inconsistencies in the consumption record.

Various devices can be used to improve quantity estimation in non-weighed records and recall methods. Food models and photos can be used to assist estimation of portion size (Moore *et al.* 1967). Household measures such as cups can be calibrated before or after use. Another suggestion has been the compilation of a photographic record to supplement the written record (Elwood & Bird 1983).

Use of food tables

All methods, apart from duplicate analysis, involve the use of food tables in order to determine the nutrient content of the diet. Food tables give a 'typical' nutrient content for unit weight of various foods 'as eaten'. It is important to realise however that these figures are only estimates. The nutrient content of any food may vary considerably depending on exactly how the food was produced and prepared and this is particularly true for the vitamins. Vitamin C content of vegetables varies with the species, the conditions of growth, the maturity, the storage time, the cooking time, the amount of water used in cooking and many other variables. In these circumstances it is not surprising to find that estimates of vitamin intake derived from food tables may differ very considerably from estimates obtained by direct analysis (Stock & Wheeler 1972; Davies, *et al.* 1973; see Chapter 9).

How long to record?

The answer to the question 'for how long should intake be recorded?' depends on the purpose of the survey. Many short records may be better than a few longer records for estimating group mean intakes. Estimation of individual intakes require records from each individual for enough days to give acceptable reproducibility.

In one dietary survey of adults in Cambridge the length of record required to classify an individual into tertiles of intake with 95% confidence was 4–5 days for energy or protein, 6–9 days for vitamin C and thiamin, 10–12 days for riboflavin and 46–64 days for vitamin A (James et al. 1983). The precise length of record required depends on the relative sizes of the variation in the day's intake within individuals and between individuals (Gardner & Heady 1973). In an American study vitamin A intake and to a lesser degree vitamin C intake were found to vary widely from day to day (Chalmers et al. 1952). This variability means that single 24 hour records are not reliable estimates of an individuals' intake though they can be used to estimate group mean intake. Recall methods are usually restricted to 24 hours because of limited memory span.

The preceding sections have discussed methods of estimating current intake but the variable relevant to nutritional status is 'habitual' or 'usual' intake. The rationale for measuring current intake is that it is believed to be an index of habitual intake though this assumption cannot be formally validated.

Short cut methods

The difficulty of measuring current intakes has stimulated attempts to develop other short cut methods of estimating habitual intake. One such method is the food frequency questionnaire which seeks to establish the 'usual' frequency and 'usual' portion size with which different foods are consumed. Estimates of nutrient intake may be made from these data. Some have suggested that even questionnaires covering very few food items may be of use in predicting nutrient intake (Hankin et al. 1968).

Burke (1947) proposed a combination of food frequency questionnaire and prospective record for assessment of nutrient intake. Food frequency questionnaires alone are probably not suitable for estimating vitamin intake in the elderly.

CONCLUSION

The extreme difficulty of obtaining reliable estimates of vitamin intake in the elderly must be borne in mind when reading reports of associations between dietary intake and biochemical indices or clinical syndromes. Probably nothing less than a seven day weighed record compiled with the aid of frequent visits from a dietitian is useful for estimating an individual's intake. Once the information on vitamin intake has been obtained, doubt about individual requirements makes it extremely difficult to interpret. It is not surprising that so much effort has been made to develop biochemical measures of nutritional status or other methods that might obviate the need to measure intake.

3 Clinical Assessment of Nutritional Status in the Elderly

W.J. MacLennan

Over the last century some of the most important advances in our understanding of human nutrition have been due to the skill of pioneers who linked clinical syndromes with specific nutrient deficiencies. Examples include the association of kwashiorkor with protein depletion, koilonychia with iron deficiency, cardiac failure with thiamin deficiency, scurvy with ascorbic acid depletion and rickets with lack of sunlight. While being indebted to the skill and perspicacity of clinicians who made these observations, we should recognise that they had the advantage of working with children and young adults where a combination of signs and symptoms was likely to be due to a single nutrient deficiency. In old people the task is more difficult in that the clinical consequences of an inadequate diet may be obscured by the effects of both multiple pathology and ageing itself. Thus an old lady with a low thiamin intake may be confused and have congestive cardiac failure, but her low thiamin intake could be because of her multi infarct dementia and her cardiac failure because of associated myocardial ischaemia.

In this situation a doctor faced with a symptom or sign said to be associated with a nutrient deficiency may check the blood level of the nutrient and finding it to be low assume that the first is the cause of the second. In reality cause and effect may be reversed, or the two findings may be coincidental. A more effective approach when confronted with a clinical abnormality is to review the wide range of nutrient deficiencies and disease states which might be responsible and embark on investigations for those which seem likely. Sometimes this process will identify a nutrient deficiency as the main cause for the problem. More usually it becomes clear that the main problem is a separate disease state, and that the nutrient deficiency is either absent or present but unrelated.

In this chapter therefore nutritional deficiency will be considered under the headings of the different tissue or organ abnormalities.

EMACIATION AND MUSCLE WASTING

It is easy to recognise a grossly emaciated elderly patient but full nutritional assessment requires quantification. Body weight can be assessed using a variety of formulas which relate weight and height (Lee *et al.* 1981). In old age however, a reduction in the thickness of intervertebral discs and kyphosis associated with osteoporosis, means that ratios based on height are of little practical value. Dehydration, which is frequently missed, is a common cause of weight loss in the elderly. When dehydration has been excluded loss of weight may be the result of fat loss or muscle wasting.

The simplest way of assessing fat loss is to use Harpenden callipers to measure the skinfold thickness at one or more sites (Jelliffe 1966; Durnin & Womersley 1974). A formula based on skinfold thickness at four sites may give a more accurate assessment of total body fat (Durnin & Womersley 1974) but this is too cumbersome for routine clinical use and has not been validated in people over the age of 75. Triceps skinfold thickness is less in those with low calorie intake than in those with normal intakes, although there is considerable overlap between the two groups especially in men (Mitchell & Lipschitz 1982).

The simplest way of assessing muscle mass is to measure the mid arm muscle circumference using the formula (Burgert & Anderson 1979):

$$\text{Arm muscle circ} = \text{Arm circ} - \frac{\pi}{10} \times \text{triceps skinfold thickness}$$
$$\qquad\quad\text{(cm)}\qquad\qquad\text{(cm)}\qquad\qquad\qquad\qquad\qquad\text{(mm)}$$

Total fat free mass can be estimated by subtracting total body fat calculated by the technique of Durnin and Womersley (1974) from total body weight. Fat free mass includes not only muscle tissue but also other tissues so it may underestimate muscle cell mass. In subnutrition changes in muscle composition can mask up to 15% muscle wasting without changing fat free mass (Heymsfield *et al.* 1982a).

Normal distributions for skinfold thickness and other anthropometric indices in the elderly have been provided by Morgan and Hullin (1982) and Burr and Phillips (1984).

While a low fat mass may be due to a reduced energy intake, it is often the result of an increased energy expenditure due to conditions such as thyrotoxicosis, Parkinson's disease, malignancy, rheumatoid arthritis and other chronic inflammatory conditions (MacLennan, *et al.* 1975). Malabsorption associated with previous gastric surgery, small bowel diverticular disease and idiopathic steatorrhoea should also be excluded (Montgomery *et al.* 1978). It is all too easy to assume that a patient with mental impairment or limited mobility has not been eating. More critical evaluation often reveals a common cause for both the mental and physical incapacity and the weight loss.

Muscle Power

Muscle power in the hand and forearm muscles may be assessed in patients who are sufficiently alert and motivated to cooperate by using a simple handgrip dynamometer (Klidjian *et al.* 1980). Tables relating means and standard deviations of grip strength to age, sex and body weight were compiled by Anderson and Cowan (1966). Ageing produces a rapid decline in grip strength while there is little change in fat free mass (Figure 3.1; MacLennan *et al.* 1980b).

When nutritional deficiency leads to proximal myopathy as it often does, measurement of grip strength is of little help. A newly developed but relatively inexpensive chair fitted with levers and strain gauges to measure the force of isometric contraction in either knee extension or elbow flexion (Maxwell *et al.* 1984) should be extremely useful in identifying muscle weakness in subnutrition, and quantifying the effect of replacement therapy.

Protein is an important source of energy, and muscle wasting therefore seems to be a useful indicator of protein or energy malnutrition (Heymsfield *et al.* 1982b). Muscle wasting due to subnutrition is associated with various functional changes (Lopes *et al.* 1982) such as weakness, delayed relaxation with consequent tendency to tetany and earlier onset of muscle fatigue.

Apart from ageing and protein deficiency, a number of other

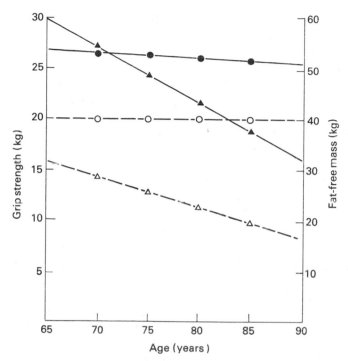

Fig. 3.1 Changes in grip strength (▲ △) and fat free mass (● ○) with age in men (——) and women (---) living at home. Note how grip strength declines rapidly while fat free mass changes very little. (MacLennan *et al.* 1980b).

factors cause muscle weakness and wasting in old age. It has long been recognised that surgery places a severe demand on nitrogen balance, and that patients with muscle wasting and hypo-albuminaemia have a high postoperative complication rate (Klidjian *et al.* 1980). Elderly patients suffer from a wide range of chronic inflammatory or malignant disorders and may have renal or liver impairment so that even if protein intake were reasonable increased catabolism might push them into negative nitrogen balance. Studies in this area are badly needed, but the practical difficulties of performing nitrogen balance studies in physically and mentally frail old people are daunting.

VITAMIN D DEFICIENCY

Many patients with osteomalacia develop a proximal myopathy (Schott & Wills 1976). Characteristic features include difficulty in getting out of a chair and a waddling gait. There is relatively little muscle wasting, no fasciculation and normal tendon reflexes. In old people more common reasons for weakened quadriceps are osteo-arthritis or immobility following an acute illness, so that there is difficulty in deciding which patients might benefit from vitamin D supplements.

Clearly patients with biochemical or radiological evidence of osteomalacia need supplementation. The approach to patients with low plasma 25-hydroxycholecalciferol levels and no other biochemical abnormalities is less obvious. Sorensen and his colleagues (1979) found that when elderly patients with osteoporosis were given 1,25-dihydroxycholecalciferol in an uncontrolled trial there was an increase in muscle enzyme activity and a rise in the number and size of fast twitch fibres. This is another area where further research might be fruitful.

ORAL CHANGES

Studies in patients with severe nutrient deficiency have demonstrated an association between oral signs and a range of vitamin and mineral deficiencies (Barker & Bender 1980). The elderly admitted to hospital are often subnourished and exhibit oral signs such as glossitis cheilitis and angular stomatitis (Table 3.1) (Brocklehurst et al. 1968), but usually the biochemical and clinical features are coincidental. In two studies treatment of elderly patients with riboflavin did not improve cheilosis or angular stomatitis. Nicotinamide had no effect on glossitis (Dymock & Brocklehurst 1973) and the administration of tablets containing riboflavin, nicotinamide, pyridoxine and ascorbic acid had no effect on tongue abnormalities (MacLeod 1972).

There has been debate about the relevance of red spots on the under surface of the tongue (figure 3.2). Initially these were considered to be small haemorrhages associated with ascorbic acid deficiency (Taylor 1966) but they were later proved to be aneurysmal dilatations of venules. It was subsequently argued

Table 3.1 Oral signs associated with nutrient deficiency.

Sign	Deficiency
Glossitis	Nicotinic acid
	Riboflavin
	Folic acid
	Vitamin B$_{12}$
Cheilosis	Riboflavin
Angular stomatitis	Riboflavin
	Iron
Sublingual petechiae	Ascorbic acid
Spongy bleeding gums	Ascorbic acid

that venular dilatation was itself due to ascorbic acid deficiency (Eddy & Taylor 1977). The evidence for this, however, is weak and treatment with ascorbic acid has no effect on their number (Andrews *et al.* 1969). The current view is that sublingual varicosities are related to age and are of little clinical importance.

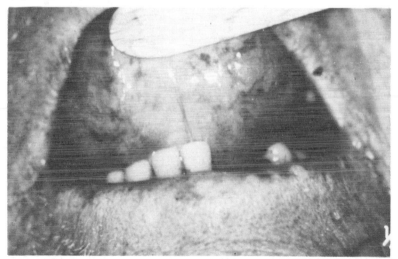

Fig. 3.2 Sublingual petechiae in an elderly patient.

SKIN CHANGES

Table 3.2 lists the more common skin changes thought to be the result of nutrient deficiency (Barker & Bender 1980). In areas where nicotinic acid deficiency is common this produces the characteristic picture of severe dermatitis and pigmentation of the face, neck, hands and other exposed surfaces. Although many old people in Britain have low intakes of nicotinic acid there is no evidence that they are more prone to dermatitis (DHSS 1972).

Table 3.2   Skin changes associated with nutrient deficiency.

Sign	Deficiency
Dermatitis	Nicotinic acid Biotin
Seborrhoeic dermatitis	Riboflavin
Hyperkeratosis	Vitamin A
Sheet haemorrhages	Ascorbic acid
Perifollicular haemorrhages	Ascorbic acid
Increased capillary fragility	Ascorbic acid

Conditions associated with hyperkeratosis including psoriasis and ichthyosis are common in old people but there is no evidence that these are associated with vitamin A deficiency or that vitamin supplements are of benefit (Ballag 1983).

ASCORBIC ACID

Elderly patients present from time to time with a classical picture of scurvy including sheet haemorrhages, brittle atrophic hairs and sheet haemorrhages in the legs. Since most are edentulous they rarely have gum sepsis or haemorrhage. They often have sheet haemorrhages on their forearms but these are due to age related changes in the connective tissue of skin and blood vessels rather than ascorbic acid deficiency (Tattersall & Seville 1950).

In contrast to scurvy, dietary and laboratory evidence of ascorbic acid deficiency is extremely common in old people (Milne *et al*. 1971), but the association between these and skin changes is tenuous. Although capillary fragility and leucocyte ascorbic acid levels are correlated, there is wide individual variation (Figure 3.3; personal observation). Tests of capillary fragility whether using a sphygmomanometer cuff or applying negative pressure are thus of little value in identifying ascorbic acid deficiency (Krasner & Dymock 1970).

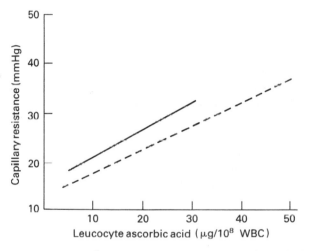

Fig. 3.3 Capillary resistance related to the leucocyte ascorbic acid concentrations in men (——) and women (-----) admitted to a geriatric unit. Capillary resistance is expressed as the negative pressure required to produce petechiae.

Evidence on the effect of ascorbic acid supplements on capillary fragility is conflicting. One study showed that patients given supplements were less likely to have a positive Hess test than controls (Brocklehurst *et al*. 1968) but another study found ascorbic acid had no greater effect than placebo in changing capillary fragility as assessed by negative pressure (Dymock & Brocklehurst 1973).

Vitamin C deficiency may be of more relevance in the situation where a patient has pressure sores or has recently undergone surgery. Vitamin C supplements certainly accelerate healing (Taylor *et al.* 1974) but it is less clear whether vitamin C deficiency is a major cause of pressure sores or delayed wound healing. Acute inflammation or trauma invariably causes a depression of leucocyte ascorbic acid levels (Figure 3.4; MacLennan & Hamilton 1977a) probably due to a dilution effect associated with leucocytosis so that it is impossible to know whether a low ascorbic acid level is due to this response or due to deficiency.

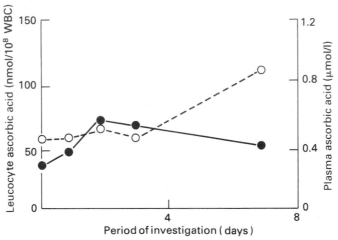

Fig. 3.4   Changes in leucocyte (○----○) and plasma (●———●) ascorbic acid concentrations in a patient recovering from bronchopneumonia. Note how recovery is associated with a rise in leucocyte ascorbic acid concentrations. (Acknowledgement of British Journal of Nutrition, MacLennan & Hamilton 1977).

ZINC

Serum zinc levels are often low in the elderly and zinc plays an important part in wound healing. It seems likely therefore that zinc deficiency is an important cause of delayed wound healing and pressure sores in this group (Busher *et al.* 1982, Sandstead *et al.* 1982). Supplements accelerate the rate of healing of surgical wounds in patients with biochemical evidence of zinc deficiency (Henzel *et al.* 1970) and may speed healing of leg ulcers (Hallbook and Lanner 1972) and pressure sores (Cohen 1968). As with ascorbic acid, catabolism associated with trauma or infection increase the utilisation of zinc so that low serum levels during infection or after injury are not always indicative of previous subnutrition (Hallbook & Hedelin 1977).

MENTAL IMPAIRMENT

Thiamin deficiency

Deficiency in B vitamins produces a variety of psychiatric abnormalities of which Wernicke's encephalopathy is the most clearly delineated (BMJ 1979). Mental symptoms include apathy, insomnia, loss of memory for recent events, disorientation and, classically, confabulation. These are often accompanied by nystagmus, occular palsies and ataxia. The condition is usually the result of alcoholism but has been reported in old people with subnutrition due to physical incapacity (Harper 1979). Few of the elderly with biochemical evidence of thiamin deficiency exhibit the classical features of Wernicke's encephalopathy (Iber *et al.* 1982) but deficiency may present with a less characteristic confusional state in high risk groups such as elderly women undergoing surgery for fractured neck of femur (Older & Dickerson 1982).

Since patients with acute confusion often show signs of subnutrition many clinicians give thiamin supplements. One regime is to inject 7 ml Parentrovite IMHP once daily for ten days. There is no firm evidence as to the efficacy of this principally because the multifactorial nature of acute confusion in the elderly makes controlled trials extremely difficult. The subject is discussed further in Chapter 7.

Nicotinic Acid deficiency

The effects of nicotinic acid deficiency on mental functioning range from headache, vertigo and insomnia to severe agitation, depression, stupor, hallucinations, confusion and convulsions and are well recognised (Bender 1980). The relevance of nicotinic acid deficiency to mental impairment in the elderly is unclear. Patients on drugs known to interfere with nicotinic acid metabolism, such as decarboxylase inhibitors and isoniazid (Bender & Smith 1978; Bender et al. 1979), may be at special risk.

Folic acid deficiency

Cases have been documented of elderly women with dementia and folic acid deficiency, whose mental function has been improved by treatment with folic acid supplements (Strachan & Henderson 1967). The deficiency is often also associated with depression (Table 3.3; Shorvon et al. 1980). Folic acid deficiency is extremely common in elderly depressed or demented patients admitted to hospital (Reynolds 1976) but generally it is the self neglect associated with the psychiatric disturbance that has caused the folate deficiency. In one trial, folic acid had no more effect than placebo on the mental function of a group of folate deficient patients with senile dementia (Shaw et al. 1971).

Table 3.3 Mental changes associated with vitamin B_{12} and folate deficiency (Shorvon et al. 1980).

	Vitamin B_{12} Deficiency		
	With pernicious anaemia (%)	Without pernicious anaemia (%)	Folate deficiency (%)
Affective disorder	19	22	56
Mental impairment	34	11	27

B_{12} Deficiency

B_{12} deficiency is also associated with both mental impairment and affective disorders. Since around 25% of patients with B_{12} deficiency have organic mental changes and 20% have depression, it is worthwhile making a psychiatric assessment of all patients with B$_{12}$ deficiency (Table 3.3; Shorvon *et al.* 1980). B$_{12}$ deficiency is a relatively rare cause of dementia. When 1004 patients aged 50 years and over admitted to a mental hospital were screened for B$_{12}$ deficiency, only two cases of pernicious anaemia were identified (Murphy *et al.* 1969). Routine measurement of serum B$_{12}$ concentrations in all elderly patients with dementia cannot be justified (see Chapter 5).

NEUROLOGICAL PROBLEMS

Spinal Cord and Peripheral Nerves

It has been recognised for many years that B$_{12}$ deficiency can produce degeneration of the peripheral nerves and of the posterior and lateral columns of the spinal cord (Walton 1982) and Table 3.4 shows the prevalence of signs associated with these lesions in patients with B$_{12}$ deficiency. Ataxia, impaired vibration and position sense, and absent tendon reflexes are all common in old age and bear little relationship to B$_{12}$ status (MacLennan *et al.* 1980). It is reasonable therefore to investigate for B$_{12}$ deficiency only if the patient also has an anaemia associated with macrocytes or polysegmented neutrophils.

Cases have been reported of patients with folate deficiency exhibiting neurological signs identical to those of B$_{12}$ deficiency which were ameliorated by folate supplements (Manzoor & Runcie 1976). Folate deficiency, however, rarely causes cord or peripheral nerve damage and in a recent series none of the 34 patients with folate deficiency had evidence of subacute combined degeneration (Shorvon *et al.* 1980). If a patient with folic acid deficiency has neurological signs, he should not be given folate supplements until after his serum B$_{12}$ concentration has been checked and shown to be normal as there is a risk of causing further neurological damage in patients who also have B$_{12}$ deficiency (Reynolds 1976).

Table 3.4 Prevalence of neurological signs in patients with vitamin B_{12} deficiency (Shorvon et al. 1980).

Signs	Vitamin B_{12} deficiency	
	With anaemia (%)	Without anaemia (%)
Distal muscle weakness	13	6
Pyramidal weakness	0	0
Ataxia (legs)	13	0
Absent ankle jerk	6	6
Areflexia (legs)	9	0
Extensor plantar reflex	22	6
Impaired vibration sense (legs)	50	22
Impaired proprioception	16	0
Impaired pain and temperature sensation	3	0
Optic atrophy	3	0

Autonomic nervous system

Ageing causes major changes in the function of the autonomic nervous system (Brocklehurst 1975; Collins et al. 1980; MacLennan et al. 1980a). Some animal experiments (Landsberg & Young 1982) suggest that nutritional deprivation could affect the sympathetic activity. Deficiencies of B vitamins might also impair autonomic function. Further research into this field is needed.

SKELETAL CHANGES

Bones are rather like the rings on a tree trunk in that their con-
figuration provides information about the life history of an individual including their nutrition. In industrial cities of Scotland
and the North of England old woman are still to be seen with
stunted growth, genu varus, tibial bowing (Figure 3.5) and
thoracic deformity, stigmata of childhood rickets resulting from
a poor diet and inadequate sunlight exposure (Paterson &
MacLennan 1984).

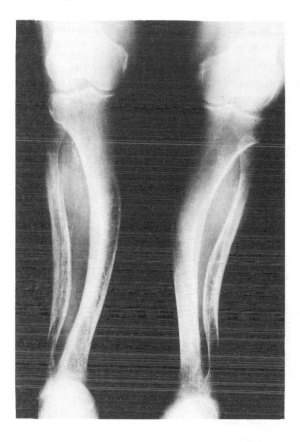

Fig. 3.5 X-Ray of tibiae of elderly woman showing deformity due to
previous rickets.

Another deformity which afflicts many old ladies is kyphos-coliosis, a condition resulting from anterior wedging of vertebral bodies generally due to osteoporosis. There is speculation as to what extent osteoporosis is the result of poor calcium nutrition. Most old people have calcium intakes well above the RDA (MacLennan et al. 1972) but the prevalence of osteoporosis may be less in areas with high calcium intakes (Matkovic et al. 1979). After the menopause the regulatory effect of oestrogens on parathyroid hormone is diminished so that the daily urinary excretion of calcium is increased (Heaney et al. 1982) and elderly women may require as much as 1.4 g of calcium per day to stay in positive balance. It remains to be seen whether the improvement in nutrition during and after World War II will reduce the pre-valence of kyphosis in old women in the future.

Kyphoscoliosis may occasionally be the result of osteomalacia and low plasma levels of 25-hydroxycholecal-ciferol are frequently found in old people. In a recent study of elderly women admitted to a geriatric unit (Wigzell et al. 1981), no correlation was found between plasma 25-hydroxycholecal-ciferol levels and the degree of kyphosis.

Other deformities of the chest wall associated with osteoporosis and osteomalacia include narrowing of the chest with flaring of the rib margins at their junction with diaphragm. Occasionally kyphosis and chest narrowing are so severe that the lower chest actually sinks into the pelvis when the patient sits and this can cause considerable discomfort.

Osteomalacia produces pelvic deformity in the young but this is rarely a problem in old age. Bone softening may cause discom-fort and pains in the pelvis and long bones are common in osteomalacia.

Deficiency of nutrients other than calcium and vitamin D can also interfere with bone synthesis. Bone formation may be sup-pressed by severe protein depletion (Jha et al. 1967). Although many old people are in negative nitrogen balance there is no evidence of a relationship between bone thickness and protein intake (MacLennan et al. 1972).

Vitamin C deficiency produces bone rarefaction in animals. Osteoporosis has been noted among South African Bantus with vitamin C deficiency induced by haemosiderosis (Lynch et al. 1967; Wapnick et al. 1971). In the elderly although both ascorbic acid deficiency and osteoporosis are common there is no evidence that the one causes the other (MacLennan *et al.* 1972; Bannerjee *et al.* 1978).

Fractured proximal femur

Bone rarefaction often manifests itself as a fracture. Above the age of 50 the incidence of fractures of the wrist rises in women possibly as a result of a postmenopausal negative calcium balance (Nordin 1980). Beginning later in life the incidence of fractures of the proximal femur also rises dramatically with age (Evans 1982). The incidence of this fracture has increased markedly (Fenton-Lewis 1981) and it is now so common that it constitutes a major public health problem. Age specific fracture rates have also been rising so that the increased incidence is only partly explained by the increasing number of elderly in the population. Non nutritional factors such as a higher frequency of falls, poor vision, dementia, cerebrovascular damage, neurological disease and general poor physical condition all contribute to the high incidence of this fracture in the elderly (Brocklehurst *et al.* 1978b). In addition to this hazards in the home environment such as poor lighting, loose rugs and unsafe furniture also contribute to the incidence of this fracture. There is some evidence, however, that nutritional deficiency (osteoporosis and osteomalacia) also predispose the elderly to fractures of the femur by causing structural weakness of the bone.

Subjects with fractured proximal femur have a lower bone mass (Cook *et al.* 1982) and more osteoporotic bone (Aaron *et al.* 1974) than controls. Most authorities accept that osteoporosis is a predisposing factor though Aitken (1984) has challenged this view. The extent to which calcium deficiency contributes to osteoporosis has been discussed earlier in this chapter. There is evidence that a change in calcium requirement after the menopause contributes to the high incidence of fractured proximal femora and this situation is exacerbated if subjects also live in areas where there is a low calcium intake (Matkovic *et al.* 1979). This highlights the importance of public health measures such as fortifying flour with calcium (Parfitt 1983).

The extent to which fractures of the hip are pointers to vitamin D deficiency is debatable. Bone biopsies from patients with proximal femoral fractures reveal thickened osteoid seams (Jenkins *et al*. 1973; Aaron *et al*. 1974; Faccini *et al*. 1976) but the histological criteria used to diagnose osteomalacia have been challenged (Hodkinson 1974). Studies based on plasma 25-hydroxycholecalciferol have given more equivocal results. Some have shown lower concentrations in fracture patients (Brown *et al*. 1976, Baker *et al*. 1979) but others have found no difference between subjects and controls (Lund *et al*. 1975, Weisman *et al*. 1978, Wooton *et al*. 1979). There is no dispute that severe vitamin D deficiency can cause fractures or that vitamin D deficiency is fairly common in the elderly population (see chapter 5). What remains to be established is whether vitamin D deficiency is an important cause of fractures in the elderly when compared with mental or physical incapacity or an inadequate calcium intake (Parfitt 1983).

Recovery of patients after they have sustained a fractured neck of femur may also be influenced by their nutritional status. Surgical patients frequently have very low intakes of food postoperatively (Hackett *et al*. 1979) and this is also true of orthopaedic patients (Hessov 1977) and of patients recovering from surgical treatment of fractured neck of femur (Older 1980). Bastow *et al*. (1983a) found that food intakes were low in patients with fracture neck of femur, and mortality was highest in the group categorised as 'very thin' who had the lowest intake. The postoperative period is a time when there is an increased protein synthesis and a high intake of protein and energy may be required to minimise protein catabolism and negative nitrogen balance. Supplementary tube feeding has been reported to be of value in reducing rehabilitation time and hospital stay in the elderly fracture patient (Bastow *et al*. 1983b).

Plasma levels of retinol are often low (Dickerson & Older 1982) and transketolase activation coefficients were raised (Older & Dickerson 1982) in patients with fractured proximal femur. These findings, however, probably reflect the acute effects of injury rather than any underlying nutritional deficiency.

CARDIOVASCULAR DISEASE

Congestive cardiac failure

The classical example of cardiac disease due to nutritional deficiency is the high output cardiac failure of thiamin deficiency (Sinclair 1982). Clinical features include a rapid pulse, a warm moist skin, raised jugular venous pressure, hepatomegaly, cardiomegaly and signs of right- or left-sided failure with flattened T waves and depressed ST segments on the ECG. Thiamin deficiency and congestive cardiac failure are both common in frail old people and though it is possible that the one sometimes exacerbates the other, the strict criteria suggested for the diagnosis of thiamin deficiency cardiac failure (Iber *et al.* 1982) are rarely met.

Ischaemic heart disease is a much more common cause of cardiac failure than thiamin deficiency. A controlled trial of thiamin supplements in thiamin deficient elderly patients with congestive cardiac failure would be difficult to organise since any effect in the few with thiamin deficient heart disease would be masked by the majority with coincidental heart disease.

Another nutritional cause of fluid retention is hypo-albuminaemia associated with protein deficiency (Fioretto & Coward 1979). Hypo-albuminaemia is common in the elderly, particularly in those with mental and physical incapacity (MacLennan *et al.* 1977) but in many elderly people with hypo-albuminaemia and oedema, the oedema is due to coincidental cardiac disease. However in a review of 1191 patients admitted to hospital by geriatricians 51 cases of oedema thought to be due to subnutrition were identified (Berry 1968). Further research into the relationship of hypo-albuminaemia and oedema in the elderly is needed.

Many old people have a low potassium intake and hypo-kalaemia is likely to occur in those taking diuretics. Potassium depletion increases the risk of developing many types of arrhythmia (MacLennan 1981). Low potassium intakes could conceivably contribute to the pathogenesis of hypertension in old age (MacGregor *et al.* 1982).

DIMINISHED RESISTANCE TO INFECTION

In childhood there is a clear association between subnutrition and increased morbidity and mortality from infection (Chandra 1983). The picture is less clear in old age where multiple pathology and ageing itself also compromise immunity. Even here, however there is mounting evidence that deficiencies of many nutrients including protein, vitamins A, E, C, and B complex may have an important effect on the response of an individual to infection. (See Chapter 7.)

Anaemia

Iron deficiency is the most common cause of anaemia in the elderly, with B_{12} deficiency occurring in about half as many subjects (Table 3.5) (MacLennan et al. 1973). Folic acid deficiency is uncommon as a cause of anaemia in old people in general, but is much more common in subgroups such as those with severe mental and physical incapacity (Read et al. 1965).

Table 3.5 Causes of anaemia in elderly patients living in the community (MacLennan et al. 1973).

Cause of anaemia	% of subjects
Iron	8
Vitamin B_{12} deficiency	4
Folate deficiency	1
Normochromic normocytic anaemia	2
Haemolytic anaemia	1

Iron deficiency

Although many old people have a low intake of iron there is no correlation between this and anaemia (MacLennan et al. 1973). In old age iron deficiency anaemia is rarely due to subnutrition and is usually the result of gastrointestinal disorders (Croker &

Banyon 1981; Walsh *et al.* 1981). Old people in good health hardly ever develop iron deficiency and anaemia (Garry *et al.* 1983).

Disorders associated with blood loss include hiatus hernia, gastric and duodenal ulcers, oesophageal varices, colonic polyps, colonic diverticula, carcinomas of stomach and colon, and haemorrhoids. A factor which complicates diagnosis in the elderly is that gastrointestinal lesions are often asymptomatic. A further problem is that conditions such as hiatus hernia, colonic diverticulae and haemorrhoids are so common in old people that the fact that they have been identified does not mean that they are the cause of anaemia.

Gastrointestinal blood loss is often the result of drug treatment (MacLennan *et al.* 1973). Before expensive hazardous and uncomfortable investigations are organised it is important to take a detailed drug history which includes details of preparations purchased direct from the pharmacist. Aspirins, indomethacin and phenylbutazone are major culprits but any of the non-steroidal anti-inflammatory agents (MacLennan *et al.* 1984) as well as the corticosteroids may be responsible for gastrointestinal ulceration or haemorrhage. Both corticosteroids and non steroidal agents are particularly likely to cause bleeding in patients who are ascorbic acid depleted, an all too common association in elderly patients with rheumatoid arthritis (Russell & Goldberg 1968).

Most clinicians rely upon a biochemical test for occult blood in faeces in order to identify gastrointestinal bleeding, but the reliability of this varies with the particular method used (Powell *et al.* 1979). This author's view is that iron deficiency in the elderly is so frequently associated with gastrointestinal blood loss that further investigations are indicated whether or not biochemical tests of the faeces support the diagnosis; the only proviso being that if the investigations are expensive, uncomfortable or hazardous they should only be performed if the patient is fit enough and likely to benefit from further medical or surgical intervention should the test results be positive.

The clinical effects of iron deficiency are difficult to define. Koilonychia is the most striking marker, but has low sensitivity while tongue signs, as discussed earlier, have low specificity in the elderly. Dysphagia associated with a pharyngeal web has been described as an effect of iron deficiency anaemia but it is no more common in anaemic patients than in controls (Elwood et al. 1964).

At one time a wide range of functional and psychological symptoms were attributed to iron deficiency. However in a controlled trial on a group of younger anaemic women iron supplements had no effect on symptoms such as headache, breathlessness, dizziness, fatigue, palpitations and irritability or on tests of psychomotor function (Elwood & Hughes 1970). In another study treatment of a group of younger anaemic patients with iron increased their maximum work capacity (Jacobs 1982), however this is only relevant to individuals with occupations involving heavy manual activity and is unimportant within the range of daily activities expected of most old people.

B_{12} Deficiency

Though B_{12} deficiency is common in old age it is rarely due to an inadequate diet (MacLennan et al. 1973). The most common cause of B_{12} deficiency is failure of intrinsic factor secretion associated with gastric atrophy. Other important, though less common conditions include previous gastric surgery, Crohn's disease of the terminal ileum and bacterial contamination associated with blind loops or small bowel diverticulae. There is also a substantial group of elderly patients who have marginally low serum B_{12} levels but whose dietary intake and absorption of B_{12} is normal (Pathy et al. 1972). A cause for their marginal deficiency has not been elucidated.

The psychiatric and neurological effects of B_{12} deficiency have been discussed (see p. 32). It is also part of medical folklore that marginal deficiency can make patients feel vaguely unwell and that B_{12} injections are effective as a tonic, however there is no clinical or psychological evidence for this proposition.

Folic acid deficiency

While folic acid deficiency is rare in healthy elderly people living at home, it is common in sick elderly people admitted to hospital, where the main factor responsible is a low dietary intake (Hurdle & Picton-Williams 1966). Detection is difficult because the serum folic acid fluctuates from day to day with dietary intake and thus is too sensitive (Raper & Chaudhury 1978). A low red cell folic acid concentration is more specific, but takes more time to develop. Raper and Chaudhury (1978) have produced evidence that elderly patients with macrocytosis often have normal serum B_{12} and red cell folate concentrations, but go on to develop florid folic acid deficiency. They suggest therefore that in the presence of a normal serum B_{12} concentration macrocytosis may be the earliest marker of folic acid deficiency.

It is essential to exclude a diagnosis of B_{12} deficiency before treating with folic acid (see p. 34).

Ascorbic acid deficiency

Most patients who have scurvy are anaemic (Goldberg 1963). Explanations for this include a disturbance of folic acid metabolism, blood loss, haemolysis and impaired iron absorption (Bender 1982). Many old people have a low ascorbic acid intake but this is usually not associated with a reduced haemoglobin concentration (MacLennan *et al.* 1973). Most old people with hypochromic anaemia respond well to iron supplements alone, but in a few resistant to this, more detailed attention to ascorbic acid deficiency might be fruitful. This is an area where more research is required.

FATIGUE, LETHARGY AND DEPRESSION

Frail elderly people suffer from a wide variety of vague and non specific symptoms. These often result from organic diseases or psychiatric neurotic or affective disorders, however deficiencies of many nutrients including potassium, iron, vitamin C, vitamin B_{12}, folate, and nicotinic acid may also contribute to the malaise. The problem is that in individual patients multiple pathology makes it difficult to disentangle the effects of subnutrition from those of physical and mental disorders. (See Chapter 5.)

DRUGS AND SUBNUTRITION

It is important to take a careful drug history from patients with subnutrition. A wide range of drugs can have important effects on nutrient metabolism and stopping an offending agent can be a lot easier than supplementing a diet with the deficient nutrient. This is one of many examples of the dangers involved in the over-enthusiastic use of drugs in the elderly (see Chapter 11).

NUTRIENT DEFICIENCIES NOT YET EVALUATED IN THE ELDERLY

Magnesium deficiency

The reason that magnesium status is often neglected by the clinician is that it is difficult to measure (Alfrey *et al.* 1974). Patients with a low serum magnesium concentration usually have a magnesium deficiency but many of those with normal concentrations may also be deficient. Information on total magnesium status can be obtained by an isotopic dilution test but equilibration of the isotope with body stores takes so long that it is little use in the clinical situation. Symptoms of depletion include convulsions, depression, vertigo, ataxia and muscular weakness (Hanna *et al.* 1960).

Ibrahim and Sutcliffe (1977) found that 44 out of 126 patients attending a geriatric day hospital had low serum magnesium concentrations. This group had symptoms which included anorexia, nausea, vomiting, confusion, tremor, tachycardia and ectopic beats, but it was not established whether these features were due to magnesium deficiency or coincident disease. Controlled trials of the efficacy of magnesium supplements are required.

Deficiency of Trace Minerals

The clinical relevance of zinc deficiency in the elderly has already been mentioned (see p. 30). Less information is available on other trace elements. The average intake of copper in the United States is very low but there is no evidence that deficiency is responsible for disease (Nordstrom 1982). Again many old people have a low intake of chromium but there is no reason to think that they suffer any disadvantage although treatment with a chromium supplement in the form of yeast produces an improvement in glucose tolerance (Offenbacher & Pi-Sunyer 1980).

A high fluoride intake may help in reducing the severity of osteoporosis (Bernstein *et al.* 1966) though it is difficult to assess the quality of bone formed. Large doses of fluoride can produce frank osteomalacia (Jowsey *et al.* 1968).

Vitamin A deficiency

The relevance of vitamin A deficiency to infection is discussed in Chapter 7 but one aspect which has received little attention is its effect on vision in the elderly. Vitamin A is essential for night vision and even mild deficiency produces an impairment in dark adaptation (Barker 1982). This is of potential importance in old age where vision is often already compromised by cataracts, glaucoma or macular degeneration and where an impaired position sense makes poor eyesight an even greater hazard.

Other vitamins

Further discussion of the effects of thiamin, nicotinic acid, pyridoxine, riboflavin and vitamin E deficiency in the elderly will be found in Chapters 4 and 5.

CONCLUSION

Despite the fact that over the past 20 years there has been a great deal of work on the intakes of nutrients and blood levels of nutrients in the elderly, this has had little impact on clinical management. We know that subnutrition is common and what causes it, but there is little information on what harm it does or whether nutritional supplements reverse the process. The main confounding factor has been that sick, elderly people are a heterogeneous group suffering from the effects of ageing, multiple pathology and polypharmacy. Further clinical research is badly needed but will only be fruitful if close attention is paid to subject selection and clinical methodology.

4   The Interpretation of Biochemical Measurements of Vitamin Status in the Elderly

D.I. Thurnham

The function of this chapter is to discuss the question 'What do biochemical measurements of vitamin status mean?' or more specifically 'Can we quantify in terms of risk the nutritional status from biochemical measurements, and if so how?'. In this book, we are particularly concerned with vitamin status in the elderly but for most vitamins, there is no distinction drawn between adults of different ages.

TESTS OF NUTRITIONAL ADEQUACY AND INADEQUACY

Brin (1964) proposed that the gradual development of a micronutrient deficiency could be divided into five stages: (1) preliminary, (2) biochemical, (3) physiological, (4) clinical and (5) morphological. Progression through the stages is dependent on the continuing presence of a deficiency and the duration and the degree of deficiency will determine the stage and the severity of signs present in an individual. This chapter will concentrate on the first two stages which are detectable only by biochemical tests but these tests are also useful in later stages of deficiency.

In the preliminary stage of a micronutrient deficiency, inadequate intake or malabsorption, or abnormal metabolism causes a reduction in tissue stores of the micronutrient. By definition at this stage the dietary intake is inadequate to maintain tissue reserves. As the deficiency continues or becomes more severe the biochemical stage is reached where modifications in metabolism can be detected. Such alterations, e.g. reduced excretion of such nutrients as riboflavin or thiamin (WHO 1967), or a fall in the concentration of tissue-bound co-enzymes (Brin 1964; Tillotson & Baker 1972), are adaptations to inadequate intake and may enable the individual to balance his metabolism and prevent further progression through the stages of deficiency. If these economies are insufficient to reduce requirements to match the inadequate intake, the deficiency will progress through the biochemical stage and eventually physiological and clinical signs will appear.

The various ways of measuring vitamin status may be grouped as follows:

1   methods which reflect the recent dietary intake. Such tests include measurement of micronutrient concentrations in plasma and micronutrient excretion in urine

2   tests more closely associated with tissue-bound vitamins and their metabolic functions (Functional tests), e.g. red cell and leucocyte concentrations, enzyme stimulation and load tests.

In general, measurements of plasma or urine levels quantify the preliminary stage while measurements in the second group quantify the biochemical and subsequent stages. Thus measurement of nutrient concentrations in body fluids can only quantify nutritional status so long as the diet is adequate. Figure 4.1 illustrates how thiamin excreted in the urine falls progressively as dietary intake of thiamin is reduced to the point where intake satisfies only the metabolic requirement at which urine thiamin tends to plateau at a basal level. When intake is less than the minimum requirement, basal concentrations of micronutrients in the plasma or excreted in the urine may be maintained by metabolic economies. Hodges *et al.* (1971) report that plasma ascorbate concentrations were maintained between 0.05 and 0.2 mg/dl for 70 days while the intake of vitamin C was zero. How long the body can maintain basal concentrations of micronutrients in the urine and plasma will depend on the availability of stored vitamins, the demand and the ability of the body to reduce its requirement. The finding of such basal concentrations of a micronutrient in body fluids tells us that the diet is inadequate, but it does not tell us for how long it has fallen below minimum requirements. Such measurements have prognostic value but they do not reflect the extent of the depletion and cannot accurately assess a subclinical or marginal deficiency state.

However enzyme activation tests and some load tests can quantify the extent of nutritional depletion. As intake of those vitamins which function as co-enzymes falls below the minimum

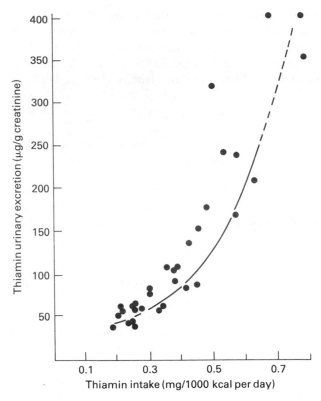

Fig. 4.1 Thiamin intake and urinary excretion. Data collected in the National Nutrition Surveys by the Interdepartmental Committee on Nutrition for National Defence (WHO 1967).

requirement, and the deficiency becomes more severe, they are progressively removed from their enzymes and increasing evidence of biochemical change can be detected. The degree of depletion is assessed by measuring enzyme activity either *in vitro* with and without the appropriate coenzyme, e.g. the enzyme stimulation tests for riboflavin, thiamin and pyridoxine (Thurnham 1981) or by administering *in vivo* substances normally metabolised by the enzyme in question, e.g. valine and histidine to assess cobalamin and folic acid status respectively (Sauberlich *et al*. 1974). Functional tests of this type are available for most of the water soluble vitamins.

Some methods for assessing status of fat soluble vitamins may also be regarded as functional tests such as the haemolysis test for vitamin E and the clotting time for vitamin K. When serum retinol or 25-hydroxycholecalciferol concentrations are low or marginal they also probably indicate the biochemical stage of deficiency.

VITAMIN DEFICIENCIES IN THE UK ELDERLY

DHSS surveys suggest that some vitamin deficiencies occurred more commonly than others (DHSS 1972; 1979a). Table 4.1 shows those vitamins which were examined in the 1973 elderly survey and the percentages of subjects found to lie in the range of values commonly associated with nutritional risk. For vitamin C, pyridoxine and folate, concentrations in both plasma and tissue were measured. For the latter 2 vitamins fewer persons were apparently at risk on the basis of the functional test than the plasma results. The vitamins for which the largest numbers of persons were nutritionally 'at risk' in 1973 were riboflavin and vitamin C. Similar results were obtained in a larger and separate survey done in 1974 (Table 4.2) in which more than 900 persons took part from 8 areas in the United Kingdom.

Table 4.1   Vitamin deficiencies in the 1973 DHSS Elderly Survey (DHSS 1979).

	163 Men (%)	193 Women (%)
Thiamin TK–AC > 1.25	8	8
Riboflavin EGR–AC > 1.30	31	30
Vitamin C PAA < 0.2 mg/dl	19	10
LAA < 15 μg/10 WBC	26	11
Pyridoxine serum PLP < 3 ng/ml	12	8
RBC PLP < 12 ng/ml	3	6
Folate serum < 3 ng/ml	13	14
RBC < 100 ng/ml	5	6
Vitamin B_{12} serum < 100 pg/ml	2	3

Table 4.2 Vitamin deficiencies in the 1974 DHSS Elderly Survey*.

	Total no.† examined	% 'at risk'
Vitamin D 25-HCC < 6 ng/ml	916	7
Thiamin TK–AC > 1.25	916	11
Riboflavin EGR–AC > 1.30	904	24
Vitamin C PAA < 0.2 mg/dl	915	31
LAA < 15 μg/10⁸ WBC	209	8

* Unpublished Survey Results.
  Subjects were drawn from 8 areas in the UK: 2 in Scotland, 1 in
  Wales and 5 in England. These areas were selected by cluster
  analysis to give as good a representation as possible of social,
  demographic, geographic and other factors relevant to elderly
  persons in the UK.
† Total number of blood samples examined was 927 (516 men, 413
  women).

    In all the DHSS surveys of the elderly it should be noted that
the participants were persons living in their own homes and
judged fit enough to cooperate in all aspects of the survey. Efforts
were made to include the full sample originally selected and the
overall results may be regarded as representative of the fitter
segment of the elderly population.

INTERPRETATION OF VITAMIN STATUS

Deficiencies of the fat soluble vitamins A, D, E and K occur less
frequently than those of the water soluble vitamins C and B complex for a variety of reasons. There may be large stores which
overcome short term deficiencies, e.g. vitamins A and D, or there
may be endogenous supplies, e.g. vitamins D and K. Dietary deficiency of vitamin E is rare. Vitamin D is the only fat soluble
vitamin whose deficiency is commonly encountered in the
elderly.

Vitamin D

The principal vitamin D metabolites found in the blood are: 25-hydroxycholecalciferol (25-HCC), 24,25-dihydroxycholecalciferol (24,25-diHCC) and 1,25-dihydroxycholecalciferol (1,25-diHCC). 25-HCC is the major metabolite and is synthesised in the liver. Further metabolism takes place in the kidney where the 1,25 or the 24,25 dihydroxy metabolites are formed according to the hormonal requirement at the time. The 1,25-diHCC stimulates calcium absorption and the restoration of serum calcium concentrations and may be the only active metabolite of vitamin D (Papaloulos *et al.* 1980). The 24,25-diHCC, however, may be required for normal bone mineralisation and structure (Weisman *et al.* 1978).

The dihydroxy metabolites are not suitable for assessing vitamin D status. The 1,25-diHCC concentration rises into the normal range on treatment with vitamin D even though the 25-HCC concentrations remain low and the 24,25-diHCC is substrate dependent and does not rise until after the 25-HCC (Papapoulos *et al.* 1980). Measurement of 25-HCC (method of Haddad and Chyu (1971)) is the most commonly used and best indicator of vitamin D status.

There are three factors to be considered when interpreting 25-HCC results in the elderly namely sex, age and time of year. Dattani *et al.* (1984) calculated separate regression lines from the DHSS 1974 survey data for 25-HCC against age for men and women in summer and winter (Figure 4.2). In all four groups 25-HCC concentrations fall with age. As the capacity to synthesise vitamin D in the skin does not fall with age (Davie & Lawson 1980) the fall in vitamin D reserves is probably due to decreasing sun exposure with increasing age.

In the elderly, 25-HCC concentration are lower in women than in men but this sex difference is not seen in children (Stamp & Round 1974; Poskitt *et al.* 1979), young adults (Stamp & Round 1974) or persons on the point of retirement (Holdsworth *et al.* 1984). Do elderly women get less sunlight exposure or are their requirements for vitamin D higher? It will be interesting to see whether the attempts of Davies and Holdsworth to teach persons at the point of retirement ways of maintaining their vitamin D levels (Holdsworth *et al.* 1984) will have any effect on their serum 25-HCC levels as they get older.

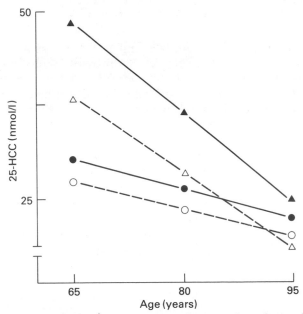

Fig. 4.2 Influence of season and sex on the relationship between
blood 25-hydroxycholecalciferol concentrations and age. (▲———▲
Males summer, △----△ Females summer, ●———● Males winter,
○----○ Females winter.) Data from the 1973 DHSS Elderly survey.
Reproduced with the authors' permission from Dattani *et al.* (1984)
Human Nutrition: Clinical Nutrition 38C, 131–7.

25-HCC values may be quoted in (nmol/l)nM or ng/ml. One
nmol/l is equal to 0.4 ng/ml.

What 25-HCC value should we accept as the threshold of deficiency? A common method of defining abnormality from a reference population is to take 2 standard deviations below the mean
as the cut off point. Holdsworth *et al.* (1984) found a range of
15–113 nmol/l (mean 55, SD 20 nmol/l) in 111 free-living adults in
the London area. Dibble *et al.* (1982) obtained a similar threshold
(12 nmol/l) from 120 samples collected throughout the year but
values less than 12 nmol/l in all patients with osteomalacia. The
latter evidence suggests that 25-HCC values below 12.5 nmol/l
represent a high risk situation for vitamin D status.

Is there a case for a higher threshold of deficiency? Lawson
et al. (1979) suggest that in order to attain concentrations of

25-HCC in the range 15–22.5 nmol/l in winter, summer values need to be above 40 nmol/l. Weisman *et al.* (1978) point out that ratios of 24,25-diHCC to 25-HCC which are invariably below normal in patients with osteomalacia were also very low in half their elderly controls whose 25-HCC concentrations were above 25 nmol/l. Possibly the elderly may require higher concentrations of 25-HCC than the young since renal impairment may well affect their ability to synthesise the dihydroxy metabolites (Aaron *et al.* 1974; Rushton 1978). It is probable therefore that concentrations of 25-HCC below 25 nmol/l should be regarded as high risk in the elderly when they occur in the months of July to October and as marginal at other times (Lawson *et al.* 1979; Dattani *et al.* 1984).

Table 4.3   Interpreting vitamin D status (25-HCC concentrations).

	nmol/l	ng/ml
High risk	< 12.5	< 5
Marginal (or high risk July–October inclusive)	12.5–25	5–10
Acceptable	> 25	> 10

Vitamin A

Vitamin A status is commonly assessed by measuring serum retinol concentrations by colorimetric or fluoromctric methods (Sauberlich *et al.* 1974). Retinol is present in the serum in a 1:1 molar combination with retinol binding protein (RBP) and circulating concentrations are tightly controlled within the normal range from 1.58–2.28 μmol/l (45–65 μg/dl) (Sauberlich *et al.* 1974). Young males tend to have slightly higher retinol (Sauberlich *et al.* 1974) and RBP (Smith *et al.* 1970) concentrations than females but no sex difference was evident in the retinol concentrations in the older age groups in the Ten State Nutrition Survey (1972).

Retinol concentrations below 0.7 μmol/l (20 μg/dl) in experimental deficiencies in man have been associated with the appearance of clinical signs of vitamin A deficiency (Hume & Krebs 1949; *et al.* 1971). Values below 0.35 μmol/l indicate a very high risk. Other factors which lower serum retinol concentrations include fever, chronic infection, liver disease, sprue, cystic fibrosis (Sauberlich *et al.* 1974) and other conditions which may impair or restrict the synthesis of RBP. Retinol is better measured in fasting blood since the concentration of circulating retinyl esters is increased directly by dietary vitamin A or indirectly from the enterohepatic circulation (Furman 1972).

Concentrations of total carotenoids and RBP and the retinol: RBP ratio have also been used to assess vitamin A status. Total carotenoids is the only method used on a regular basis but reflects only the dietary intake of carotenoids. RBP gives the same information as serum retinol but has the advantage that it can be measured on 20 μl of serum (LC Partigen immunodiffusion plates, Hoechst). The serum retinol: RBP ratio may be of some additional use in interpreting serum retinol values. In deficiencies of vitamin A, the molar ratio falls due to the accumulation of apo-RBP (Glover *et al.* 1974) and may be elevated in hypervitaminosis A due to the presence of free retinyl esters (Smith & Goodman 1976).

Table 4.4   Interpreting vitamin A status.

	Retinol and total carotenoids μmol/l	Retinol μg/dl	Total carotenoids μg/dl
High risk	< 0.35	< 10	< 20
Medium risk	0.35–0.7	10–20	20–40
Acceptable	> 0.7	> 20	> 40

Vitamin E

Vitamin E deficiency is rare in humans and apart from some newborn infants (Gross 1976) it is only likely to occur in some cases of fat malabsorption (Tomasi 1979). There are 8 naturally occurring compounds with vitamin E activity (Piironen *et al.* 1983) but α-tocopherol is predominant in the blood and total vitamin E activity is usually measured to assess vitamin E status. The haemolysis test originally proposed by Rose & Gyorgy (1952) to assess the stability of red cells in the presence of dilute hydrogen peroxide may also be used. The methods available for measurement of vitamin E status have recently been reviewed by Desai (1980). The requirement for vitamin E is a function of the tissue content of polyunsaturated fatty acids and hence the ratio of vitamin E to lipid in the serum in a better measure of status than serum vitamin E alone (Horwitt *et al.* 1972). Thresholds to interpret these 3 methods are illustrated in Table 4.5.

Table 4.5   Interpreting vitamin E status.

	Serum vitamin E		Haemolysis test (%)	Vitamin E: total lipid ratio (mg/g)
	μmol/l	mg/dl		
High risk	< 1.16	< 0.5	> 20	< 0.8
Medium risk	1.16–1.63	0.5–0.7	10–20	not defined
Acceptable	> 1.63	> 0.7	< 10	> 0.8

Vitamin K

Vitamin K is required in man to maintain prothrombin and other factors (VII, IX and X) necessary for normal blood clotting. Deficiency of vitamin K is rare but may occur in patients with diseases affecting the metabolism or absorption of vitamin K, in patients receiving drugs such as antibiotics which interfere with intestinal vitamin K synthesis or such as anticoagulants which interfere with prothrombin synthesis (Sauberlich *et al.* 1974).

The clinical manifestation of vitamin K deficiency is haemorrhage as a result of delayed blood clotting. Tests which measure overall clotting kinetics such as the Quick one-stage prothrombin time test (Quick 1970) provide a rapid and inexpensive way of measuring vitamin K status. Hazell and Baloch (1970) used this test on 1,110 elderly patients and found prolonged prothrombin times in nearly 75% of those studied. Oral vitamin K normalised the response in most of the patients. The result serves to draw attention to the vitamin K status in the elderly since most of the patients were found to have hepatic damage or to be taking drugs with anticoagulant action.

Vitamin C

Methods to assess vitamin C status have recently been reviewed (Sauberlich *et al.* 1974; Sauberlich 1975). The two main methods are the measurement of plasma (PAA) and buffy layer vitamin C (BAA) concentrations. BAA is considered to be a measure of tissue stores, while plasma reflects recent dietary intake. Unfortunately the buffy layer measurement requires a large amount of blood and has to be processed fairly quickly before the leucocytes can take up vitamin C from the plasma (Denson & Bowers 1961). In elderly subjects we found a reasonably good correlation between these two methods (men r = 0.46, p < 0.001; women r = 0.32, p < 0.001: DHSS 1979a) confirming Burr *et al.* (1974a). The plasma assay gives sufficient information to assess vitamin status in population studies but great care must be exercised in interpreting low values.

Table 4.6 Relationship between the intake and serum concentration of vitamin C.

Intake (mg/day)	PAA (mg/dl)*
< 7	0.20
8	0.18
< 10	< 0.10
10–29	< 0.20
23	0.20
25	0.29
32	0.48
33	0.47
57	0.72
58	0.74
75	0.84
82	0.93
83	1.47
107	1.05
133	1.69

* Individual reports compiled by Sauberlich *et al.* (1974)

Table 4.6 shows the near linear relationship between dietary vitamin C intake and PAA over the concentration range 17–80 μmol/l (0.3–1.4 mg/dl). Similar data have been reported by Newton *et al.* (1983). The plateau PAA value of 80 μmol/l is reached at an intake of about 100 mg/day. At higher intakes the body tissues are saturated and urinary excretion of unchanged vitamin increases rapidly. Deprivation studies show that with very low intakes PAA fluctuates between 6 and 17 μmol/l unrelated to intake (Hodges *et al.* 1971). PAA values between 17 and 80 μmol/l are probably reliable indicators of dietary intake but below this range the relationship breaks down. PAA values in the range 6–17 μmol/l do not necessarily indicate imminent scurvy, although scurvy can appear at this level. Values of PAA below 6 μmol/l indicate a very high nutritional risk, but they are on the limits of sensitivity of the assay and should be confirmed by a BAA measurement. PAA is thus primarily a measure of the preliminary stage of deficiency and low values only indicate that the diet is poor.

The normal range reported for BAA was 148–199 pmol (26–35 μg)/10^8 WBC in young adults (Denson & Bowers 1961; Bowers & Kubic 1965). Windsor and Williams (1970) proposed that the lower limit of acceptability in elderly persons was 86 pmol (15 μg)/10^8 WBC and they found evidence to suggest that proline metabolism may be impaired below this BAA concentration. During dietary deprivation BAA declines more slowly than PAA and only approaches zero with the onset of scurvy (MRC 1948; Bartley *et al.* 1953). Values of BAA less than 40 pmol/10^8 WBC occur when body stores are depleted and indicate a high risk of vitamin C deficiency. Guidelines for interpreting vitamin C status are summarised in Table 4.7.

Table 4.7 Interpreting vitamin C Status.

	Serum vitamin C		Buffy layer Vitamin C	
	μmol/l	mg/dl	pmol/10^8 WBC	μg/10^8 WBC
High risk	< 6	< 0.1	< 40	< 7
Medium risk	6–17	0.1–0.3	40–86	7–15
Acceptable	> 17	> 0.3	> 86	> 15

Although BAA is a better indicator of vitamin C status, it does represent 2 blood components which may vary independently, i.e. the platelets and the leucocytes. In the normal person, platelets and leucocytes contribute equally to the total vitamin C content. Following surgery there is a fall in platelets and an increase in leucocytes with the net effect that the BAA falls (Coon 1962; Evans *et al.* 1980).

Both PAA and BAA are usually lower in men than women (Sauberlich *et al.* 1974) and both may be lower in oral contraceptive users (Briggs & Briggs 1972; Harris *et al.* 1973) although others do not confirm this (Horwitt *et al.* 1975; Yeung 1977). It has also been reported that PAA and BAA tend to be lower in elderly subjects (Kirk & Chieffi 1953a; 1953b; Andrews & Brook 1966; Griffiths *et al.* 1967) though Garry *et al.* (1982) did not find this.

Thiamin

Thiamin status is usually measured by the transketolase assay which is a functional test based on the fact that thiamin pyrophosphate is the co-enzyme essential for transketolase activity. Transketolase activity in a red cell haemolysate is measured without (basal) and with (stimulated) added thiamin pyrophosphate (TPP). The result may be expressed either as transketolase activation coefficient (TK–AC), the ratio of stimulated to basal activity or as TPP effect (%), the difference between stimulated and basal activity as a percentage of basal (Brin *et al.* 1960). The experimental removal of thiamin from the diet reduces the red cell transketolase activity but this loss of activity can be partially replaced *in vitro* by addition of TPP and incubation results in an increased TPP effect.

TPP effect may be measured either by a colorimetric assay such as that of Schouten *et al.* (1964) or by a rate reaction technique originally described by Smeets *et al.* (1971). The colorimetric method overestimates transketolase activity and underestimates TPP effect due to a basic defect in the general technique (Warnock 1976) and has the further disadvantages of lengthy colour development and corrosive reagents. The rate reaction technique avoids all these problems but the low enzyme activity in the face of a high background absorbance from haemoglobin makes measurement difficult and quenches NAD absorbance although the latter may be corrected (Buttery *et al.* 1980).

A general problem of all transketolase assays is that the enzyme is unstable *in vitro* and has to be analysed reasonably quickly (Vo-Khactu *et al.* 1974; Bayoumi & Rosalki 1976). Furthermore the apoenzyme is unstable *in vivo* so that in long-standing deficiency the TPP effect may not be so high as to reflect the full severity of the deficiency, and measurement of absolute enzyme activity is necessary to assess the full extent of the thiamin deprivation. Some Australian workers (Wood *et al.* 1977) maintain that basal transketolase activity is a better measure of thiamin deficiency than TPP effect though measurements of TPP effect are more easily standardised for inter-laboratory comparisons (Vo-Khactu *et al.* 1974).

Brin (1962) originally proposed that a TPP effect above 15% (TK–AC > 1.15) indicated thiamin deficiency and above 25% (TK–AC > 1.25) severe deficiency. Many workers have only accepted TPP effect above 25% as indicating deficiency (Chong & Ho 1970; Bayoumi & Rosalki 1976). The author knows of no reports where sex or age influence the assay although some drugs such as 5-fluorouracil (Basu, *et al.* 1979) and frusemide (Yui *et al.* 1980) may impair thiamin status. A reticulocytosis increases transketolase activity and may lower the TPP effect (Wells & Marks 1972). Table 4.8 summarises the interpretation of the transketolase test.

Table 4.8 Interpreting thiamin status*.

	TK–AC	TPP effect (%)
†High risk	> 1.25	> 25
Marginal risk	1.11–1.25	11–25
Acceptable	< 1.11	< 11

† Because of difficulties with the assay some workers believe that a risk can only be attached to values > 1.25 and that all values < 1.25 are acceptable.

* Enzyme activity can also be used to assess status but individual laboratories must establish their own reference ranges.

Riboflavin

The principal method now used to assess riboflavin status is the red cell stimulation test in which erythrocyte glutathione reductase is assayed with and without flavin adenine dinucleotide (Glatzle *et al.* 1968; Bamji 1969; Beutler 1969) and the ratio of these activities is termed the activation coefficient (EGR–AC). It is a functional test and the principle is the same as that described for thiamin. Glutathione reductase differs from transkotolase in that it is very stable *in vitro* (Thurnham & Rathakette 1982) and the high EGR–AC values obtained in some developing countries (Bates *et al.* 1981; Thurnham *et al.* 1982) would suggest that the apoenzyme is also very stable *in vivo*.

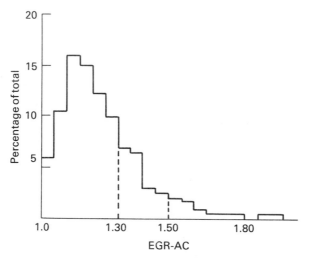

Fig. 4.3   Distribution of EGR-AC, a measure of riboflavin status in the elderly. Data from the 1973 and 1974 DHSS Elderly surveys combined. Of the 1 333 elderly subjects examined 32% (133/416) and 26% (237/917) in the two surveys respectively had EGR-AC > 1.30.

Figure 4.3 shows a histogram of the combined EGR–AC values obtained in the 1973 and 1974 DHSS surveys of the elderly. About 30% of all the elderly persons lay in the deficient range (EGR–AC > 1.3). There was no difference between the sexes or age groups confirming the findings of others (Nichoalds *et al.* 1974). Apart from nutrition the stimulation test is only disturbed by factors affecting red cell synthesis or metabolism (Nichoalds *et al.* 1974; Thurnham 1981).

Glatzle *et al.* (1970) proposed an upper limit of normal of 1.2 on the grounds that all EGR–AC values in a group of elderly people fell below this level after supplementation with riboflavin. Modifications to the original method such as the order of adding reagents seem to give slightly higher results. Most workers now take 1.3 as the upper limit of normal (Tillotson & Baker 1972) although a few still use a lower limit while Bayoumi and Rosalki (1976) use 1.76.

The choice of 1.3 is supported by figure 4.4 which shows regression lines and correlation coefficients of EGR–AC on dietary riboflavin intake (men $r = -0.25$, women $r = -0.29$) from the 1973 DHSS survey of the elderly. Distribution of the data was wide and the dietary intakes only explain about 14% of the variance in the biochemical values, but at the intake equivalent to minimum daily requirement the EGR–AC value in both sexes is very close to 1.3 suggesting that this is an appropriate upper limit. The community studies of Bates *et al.* (1982) in the Gambia show that EGR–AC values between 1.5 and 1.8 are

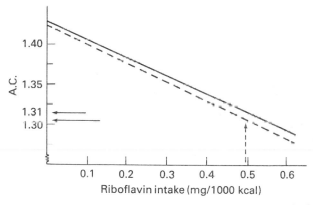

Fig. 4.4 Regression lines for EGR-AC, a measure of riboflavin status on riboflavin intake for subjects in the 1973 DHSS Elderly Survey (DHSS 1979). Men (166, ———); and women (192, ---) are represented separately on the graph.

associated with very low riboflavin intakes of 0.5 mg/day. Tillotson and Baker (1972) suggested that EGR–AC greater than 1.8 should be regarded as severely deficient.

Clinical evidence of riboflavin deficiency in communities where higher EGR–AC values (> 1.3) occur is usually poorly correlated with the biochemical status (Thurnham *et al*. 1971; Bates *et al*. 1982) though there are some haematological changes associated with EGR–AC values > 1.3 (Powers & Thurnham 1981). Acute deprivation studies also show little correlation between clinical signs and EGR–AC values (Tillotson & Baker 1972). Criteria for evaluating riboflavin status based on EGR–AC values are summarised in Table 4.9.

Table 4.9   Interpreting riboflavin status*.

	EGR–AC
High risk	> 1.8
Medium risk	1.5–1.79
Low risk	1.3–1.49
Acceptable	< 1.29

* Applies to those methods which start the reaction using NADPH

Vitamin B$_6$

Vitamin B$_6$ or pyridoxine is coenzymatically active as pyridoxal-5-phosphate (PLP) which is intimately associated with amino acid metabolism in the body. Deficiencies of this vitamin are rare but experimentally the effects are diverse and have been reported to provoke changes in many tissues including the nervous, blood forming, vascular and skin.

Many ways have been proposed for the assessment of pyridoxine status. These include: (1) measurement of plasma PLP concentration, (2) a functional test analagous to that used for thiamin in which red cell apartate aminotransferase (AST) is measured with and without PLP to give an activation coefficient

(AST–AC), (3) the tryptophan loading test (4) measurement of urinary PLP and (5) measurement of urinary 4-pyridoxic acid (Sauberlich *et al.* 1974).

It has been known for some time that plasma PLP concentrations were lower in the elderly than younger members of the population. Hamfelt (1964) found a mean value of 13.8 nmol/l (3.4 ng/ml) in 20 healthy elderly people compared with means of 28, 45 and 65 nmol/l in progessively younger age groups. In 11 of these elderly people with low PLP values the tryptophan loading test showed a high excretion of xanthurenic acid thus indicating a deficiency of vitamin B_6. No data was given for those with higher PLP values, however, nor was an attempt made to correlate the individual results of the two tests. The loading test has recently fallen into disrepute since it has been shown to be affected not only by pyridoxine status, but also by hormonal changes particularly of oestrogen (Wynick & Bender 1981). It is unlikely that hormonal changes could explain Hamfelt's results in the elderly subjects, but nevertheless, results from the tryptophan loading must be interpreted carefully.

Anderson *et al.* (1970) confirmed the fall in PLP with age using a microbiological method which measures both PLP and pyridoxal. Pyridoxal represents some 20–60% of the pyridoxine vitamers in the plasma (Chauhan & Dakshinamurti 1979). Despite the different method they too obtained many low values in elderly subjects and a mean value only marginally higher than that of Hamfelt namely 21.5 nmol/l. To what extent the low plasma PLP values in the elderly are due to dietary as opposed to physiological factors, is unclear. Anderson clearly felt that the fall was chiefly physiological since she adopted 12 nmol/l as the lower limit of normal for the elderly (DHSS 1979a).

Singkamani (unpublished work) investigated the relationship between plasma PLP and the red cell AST stimulation assay in patients aged 16–98 admitted for minor operations to Dudley Road Hospital, Birmingham. Plasma PLP declined with age but the AST indices did not correlate with age. Mean concentration of plasma PLP in 49 patients aged more than 60 years was 27.0 nmol/l and 18 of them (37%) had plasma PLP less than 12 nmol/l. There was no correlation between plasma PLP and basal red cell AST activity or AST–AC values, although there was a very close correlation between basal AST activity and

AST–AC values. Plasma PLP originates in the liver (Lumeng et al. 1974). Plasma PLP rises rapidly after a dose of vitamin B_6 (Contractor & Shane 1968) and so reflects recent dietary intake of the vitamin. The metabolism of pyridoxine may also be different in the elderly since the lower concentration of plasma PLP may be associated with increased catabolism to 4-pyridoxic acid (see Sauberlich et al. 1974). The complete lack of correlation between plasma PLP and AST–AC suggests that more work is needed to determine the relevance of these tests as measures of pyridoxine status in the elderly.

To conclude, the red cell stimulation test (AST–AC) may prove to be the best assay of pyridoxine status. The measurement is straightforward, sensitive and unrelated to age. Unfortunately a large number of modifications of the basic method exist and the interpretation has not yet been standardised. A threshold somewhere between 1.5 and 2.0 is probably the upper limit of normal, and tentative criteria to interpret pyridoxine status are shown in Table 4.10. For a fuller discussion consult Sauberlich et al. (1974).

Table 4.10   Interpreting pyridoxine status.

	Plasma PLP		Red cell PLP		Stimulation test
	nmol/l	ng/ml	nmol/l	ng/ml	AST–AC
Nutritional risk	< 12	< 3	< 49	< 12	> 2.0
Marginal risk	12–16	3–4	49–57	12–14	1.5–2.0
Acceptable	> 16	> 4	> 57	> 14	< 1.5

Folacin

The two most useful methods for assessing folate status are the measurements of serum and red cell folacin concentrations. White cell folacin concentrations correlate well with red cell folacin but the method has no practical advantages. The histidine load test in which the urinary excretion of formiminoglutamic acid (FIGLU) is examined is of practical use only in clinical situations (Sauberlich et al. 1974).

Red cell and serum folacin measurements have been reported to correlate well (Hoffbrand *et al.* 1966) although they indicate different aspects of folate nutriture. Experimental studies in man have shown that serum folate falls very rapidly on folate deficient diets to values less than 3 ng/ml after 22 days while red cell folate fell much more slowly and low values (< 200 ng/ml) were only seen after 123 days on the diet (Herbert 1967). Both measurements therefore are good indicators of folate status but serum folate reflects the dietary intake and more readily available tissue reserves, while a low red cell folate is more serious, indicating a more long-standing deficiency. Thresholds to interpret results from the two methods are shown in Table 4.11.

Table 4.11 Interpreting folate and vitamin B_{12} status.

	Serum folate		RBC folate		Serum B_{12}	
	nmol/l	ng/ml	mmol/l	ng/ml	pmol/l	pg/ml
Nutritional risk	< 6.8	< 3	< 0.23	< 100	< 74	< 100
Marginal	6.8–13.4	3.0–5.9	0.23–0.34	100–150	74–147	100–200
Acceptable	> 13.4	> 5.9	> 0.34	> 150	> 147	> 200

Folate status is correlated with vitamin C status (DHSS 1979a) and it has been suggested that low vitamin C status in the elderly may impair folate metabolism. However the low vitamin C status of the elderly in the DHSS survey would not appear to be the cause of the low folate values since vitamin C supplementa tion over two months failed to influence plasma folate status even in those with low vitamin C status at the start (Bates *et al* 1980).

Vitamin B$_{12}$

Vitamin B$_{12}$ status is estimated from the concentrations of the vitamin in the serum (Table 4.11). In the 1973 DHSS survey of the elderly approximately 2.5% of both sexes were in the deficient range (< 100 pg/ml). A further 15% of men and 20% of women lay within the marginal range of 100–200 pg/ml. The overall mean value for serum B$_{12}$ was lower than those obtained for younger people. The subject is further discussed in chapter 5.

Nicotinic acid

Nicotinic acid status is assessed by measuring the urinary metabolism N^1-methyl-nicotinamide (NMN) and N^1-methyl-2-pyridone-5-carboxamide (2-pyridone). NMN accounts for 20–30% and 2-pyridone 40–60% of the total nicotinic acid metabolites present in urine. The ratio of NMN to 2-pyridone in the normal individual is in the range 1.3–4.0 and ratios less than 1.0 indicate deficiency.

The urinary concentration of 2-pyridone falls rapidly on a nicotinic acid deficient diet and reaches zero many weeks before clinical deficiency appears while the concentration of NMN falls more gradually as the deficiency progresses. Urinary NMN is thus a better indicator of nicotinic acid status than 2-pyridone but the best indicator is the ratio of the two metabolites as it overcomes variations in the amounts of the individual metabolites excreted in different populations (Sauberlich et al. 1974). Thresholds for interpretation of nicotinic acid status are summarised in Table 4.12.

Other Vitamin deficiencies

Only two other vitamins need to be mentioned. Pantothenic acid is a component of co-enzyme A and participates in numerous important biochemical reactions but is ubiquitous in nature and dietary deficiency is most unlikely. Biotin is also an essential cofactor in numerous enzymes but its deficiency has only rarely been reported and usually in conjunction with the consumption of excessive amounts of raw egg white.

Table 4.12 Interpreting nicotinic acid status.

	N^1-methyl-nicotinamide*		
	mg/g creatinine	mmol/mol creatinine	Ratio**
Nutritional risk	< 1.5	< 1.24	< 1.0
Marginal	1.6–4.29	1.32–3.54	
Acceptable	> 4.9	> 3.54	1.0–4.0

* These figures apply to adults: males, non-pregnant and non-lactating females only.

** Ratio of NMN to 2-pyridone. Applicable to all persons under most circumstances (Sauberlich *et al.* 1974).

5 The Prevalence of Vitamin Deficiency in the Elderly

M.L. Burr

Prevalence implies a numerator and a denominator, the latter being the population at risk, while the former is the number of cases of the condition within that population. The prevalence of vitamin deficiency is estimated from the results of dietary, biochemical and clinical surveys. In some surveys the subjects were clearly atypical of old people in general, while in others the response-rate was so low (below 70%) that those who were seen cannot be assumed to represent the whole sample. In such surveys the denominator is not adequately represented, and the prevalence is consequently uncertain.

The numerator also presents problems. Before the cases of vitamin deficiency can be counted, the condition must be defined in terms of intake, biochemistry or clinical signs, and agreement is still largely lacking on these criteria. An indirect approach is the prospective study, in which persons of known vitamin status are followed up. If there is no detectable difference in outcome between sufficient persons with a wide range of vitamin status it may reasonably be concluded that no part of that range constitutes deficiency. Unfortunately an association between a low vitamin status and mortality or morbidity is ambiguous. Vitamin deficiency may have caused the poorer outcome, or ill-health and premature ageing may have affected both the low vitamin status and the prognosis. Clearer evidence is derived from randomised controlled trials of vitamin supplementation, which address the question 'What proportion of elderly people would benefit from a higher intake of this vitamin?'

VITAMIN C

The mortality attributed to vitamin C deficiency is very low in developed countries. In 1982 there was only one death registered as due to scurvy in England and Wales. Yet frank scurvy does occur, sometimes it is diagnosed and treated, and other times it remits spontaneously following a change in diet.

Dietary Intake

Four British dietary surveys have found group mean intakes of vitamin C of 32–46 mg per day in elderly men and 27–40 mg per day in elderly women (MacLeod *et al.* 1974; Lonergan *et al.* 1975; DHSS 1972, 1979a). These figures do not include supplementary vitamins, which are taken by about 6.6% of old people in Britain if all vitamin supplements are included (DHSS 1979a). Vitamin C intakes are lower in women than in men, and particularly low in Scotland, where 5% of the elderly have been found to take less than 10 mg per day (MacLeod *et al.* 1974). The dietary vitamin C intake of old people in Vancouver is about twice the above levels (Leichter *et al.* 1978). It is possible that adaptation to a low intake may occur if it continues for a long time. In Africa and India high blood levels have been reported in persons with intakes of 10 mg or even less per day (Andersson *et al.* 1956; Rajalakshmi *et al.* 1965; Srikantia *et al.* 1970). There is also some evidence of adaptation to a high intake, including a higher rate of catabolism of vitamin C if it continues for a long time (Schrauzer & Rhead 1973; Sorensen *et al.* 1974).

Blood concentrations

Ascorbic acid can be measured in the plasma and the leucocytes. In various surveys mean plasma levels have been reported of 0.2–0.5 mg/dl in men and 0.4–0.6 mg/dl in women, mean leucocyte levels being 14–23 and 19–26 μg/10^8 cells respectively (Milne *et al.* 1971; DHSS 1972, 1979a; Burr *et al.* 1974a). There is some evidence that plasma ascorbate is lower in older than in younger people even if their intake is the same, possibly due to impaired absorption (Kirk & Chieffi 1953; Burr *et al.* 1974b). Elderly Asian immigrants tend to have a low serum ascorbate compared with other old people in the same English town (Elwood *et al.* 1972). Men who live alone have a lower leucocyte ascorbate than other men, but in women the situation is reversed, and those who live alone have higher values (DHSS

1972; Burr, et al. 1982b). Presumably the women have been cooking meals for most of their lives and care for themselves even better when they live alone than before.

Clinical surveys

In the two surveys conducted by the Department of Health and Social Security (1972, 1979a) frank scurvy was diagnosed in two out of 879 subjects (0.2%), and in 3 out of 365 (0.8%) respectively. Some surveys have included an assessment of minor signs which, in association with other evidence, may indicate marginal vitamin C deficiency. Among patients in hospital a low vitamin C status is often associated with sublingual haemorrhages (Andrews & Brook 1966; Taylor 1968), which are absent among elderly vegetarians with a high vitamin C status (Eddy & Taylor 1977). In the second DHSS (1979a) survey sublingual varicosities (but not haemorrhages) were associated with a low leucocyte concentration.

Prospective studies

Three studies examined the short-term prognostic significance of blood ascorbate in patients admitted to acute geriatric wards. In two of these a low leucocyte ascorbate concentration tended to predict death within four weeks (Wilson et al. 1972, 1973); in the third, plasma ascorbate was unrelated to outcome (Kemm & Allcock 1984). In another hospital study leucocyte ascorbate below 15 μg/10^8 WBC was associated with higher mortality within 24 weeks (Hunt et al. 1984). Long-term studies suggest that intake of vitamin C (Hodkinson & Exton-Smith 1976), or its concentration in plasma and leucocytes (Burr et al. 1975, Burr, et al. 1982a), continues to predict mortality after several years. It is by no means clear, however, whether these associations imply that a low vitamin C status actually contributed to risk of death.

Randomised trials

Several controlled trials have been conducted in which old people have received vitamin C supplements or matching placebo tablets. Three studies examined the effect of vitamin C on mortality (Wilson *et al.* 1973; Burr, *et al.* 1975; Hunt *et al.* 1984) and none of them revealed any significant effect. Furthermore, no effect was detected on the incidence of illnesses and mental function in the second of these trials or on clinical progress in the third. The trial by Andrews *et al.* (1969) failed to show any effect of vitamin C on sublingual lesions, and that by MacLeod (1972) showed no effect of multivitamin supplements on tongue signs or angular stomatitis. On the other hand, two trials by Schorah *et al.* (1979, 1981) showed small gains in weight and slight clinical improvement in long-stay patients receiving vitamin C in comparison to others receiving matched placebo tablets. Another controlled trial (Taylor *et al.* 1974) suggested that vitamin C supplements may promote the healing of pressure sores.

The most striking evidence for widespread vitamin deficiency was provided by the Farnborough trial (Taylor 1968). Eighty long-stay inpatients were randomly allocated to receive either a multivitamin supplement, (including 200 mg vitamin C daily) or a matched placebo. The patients were examined regularly by a physician, who successfully detected all those receiving the vitamin supplement by 12 months.

Comment

There is no agreed definition of vitamin C deficiency in terms of dietary intake, biochemical status or clinical signs. It is therefore not possible to determine its prevalence, except for frank scurvy, which has been found in 0.2–0.8% of elderly subjects in the DHSS surveys. Nearly half the old people in Britain take less than 30 mg daily (the British recommended daily intake), but there is no clear evidence that they would benefit from a higher intake. It is possible that adaptation occurs to a long-continued high or low intake, so that a given diet may imply deficiency for one person but not for another. There is also evidence that the absorption or metabolism of vitamin C differs slightly between men and women (men having higher intakes but lower plasma and leucocyte levels than women), and between old and young subjects (the elderly having lower plasma levels for a given intake). It may therefore be inappropriate to search for a single optimum intake that applies to everyone.

Most of the prospective studies suggest that vitamin C status predicts mortality, though randomised controlled trials show no effect of vitamin supplementation on death-rates or disease incidence. This apparent discrepancy can be explained in several ways. The controlled trials might have been too small, or perhaps the effect of vitamin C deficiency is irreversible, so that it is too late to give old people vitamin C and expect to see any improvement. It may be that people in poor health and consequential increased risk of death do not eat as well as their healthier contemporaries, and therefore have a low vitamin C status.

Nevertheless there is some evidence, derived from controlled trials, that some old people would derive small benefits to general health from taking more vitamin C. It seems likely that many inpatients in long-stay wards have some impairment in the ability of small blood vessels to heal, and this can be improved by vitamins, particularly vitamin C.

It therefore seems reasonable to conclude that minor degrees of vitamin C deficiency do exist in addition to overt cases of scurvy, especially among old men living alone and long-stay hospital inpatients, but the prevalence cannot be determined in the absence of clear criteria for diagnosis.

VITAMIN D

In 1982 there were sixteen deaths in England and Wales attributed to vitamin D deficiency. Obviously this figure gives no indication of the prevalence of the condition, especially since it is not always looked for in cases in which it may have contributed to illness or death.

$$1\mu g \equiv 40 \, iu.$$

Dietary intake and sunlight

The mean dietary intake of vitamin D for elderly British people is about the level (2.5 μg/day) recommended by the Department of Health (DHSS 1972, 1979a; MacLeod et al. 1974; Lonergan et al. 1975). Men have a higher intake than women and there is no consistent relationship with age. A low intake is not synonymous with deficiency since adequate exposure to sunlight will provide sufficient vitamin D without any dietary intake. Many authorities (Hodkinson *et al.* 1973; Lawson *et al.* 1979; Fraser 1983) consider that sunlight is more important than diet in providing vitamin D in the elderly, but this view has recently been questioned (Sheltawy *et al.* 1984). There are reasons for believing that the body is better adapted to handle vitamin D which is derived from sunlight, than that which is absorbed from food (DHSS 1980). It seems that vitamin D is transferred from the skin to the blood at a controlled rate, whereas by mouth it is more rapidly absorbed and less well conserved, thus giving rise to wide fluctuations in plasma 25-hydroxycholecalciferol (Fraser 1983).

It is possible that some old people need a higher intake of vitamin D in the absence of sunlight than do younger people. Skylab astronauts (who received no sunlight) required 10 μg vitamin D daily to maintain plasma 25-HCC levels. But in a group of housebound elderly persons 25 μg was needed to raise plasma levels in all subjects (references in Parfitt *et al.* 1982). On the other hand, in another study (Johnson *et al.* 1980) 50 μg vitamin D per day caused hypercalcaemia in two out of 63 elderly persons. This is disturbing since the margin between the physiological and the toxic dose of vitamin D is usually assumed to be very wide. It may be that some old individuals are especially sensitive to vitamin D, so that the safety margin may be narrow in the elderly.

Blood Levels

In view of the variable contribution made by sunlight, vitamin D status is more appropriately assessed by plasma 25-hydroxycholocalciferol levels than by dietary intake. The lower limit of normality is discussed in Chapter 4 and old people in Britain frequently have values below 25 nmol (10 ng/ml). Thus in a survey of 916 subjects over the age of 65 years living in their own homes, the mean plasma 25-HCC values in summer for men and women respectively were 16.2 and 13.1 ng/ml and in winter the mean values were 11.1 and 9.9 ng/ml respectively (Dattani *et al.* 1984). Lower concentrations were reported by Corless *et al.* (1975) in long-stay geriatric patients. They found that 36 patients who never went out of doors had a median 25-HCC concentration of

1.3 ng/ml, while 9 patients who sometimes went outside had a median concentration of 4.3 ng/ml.

In the UK rickets and osteomalacia seem to occur in persons of Asian descent far more often than in the indigenous population. Suggested explanations for this include skin pigmentation, genetic factors, dietary insufficiency of vitamin D, dietary excess of phytate (especially in chapattis), and inadequate exposure to sunlight. Comparative studies among Asian people living in India and in Britain suggest that it is the difference in exposure to sunlight that is the most important factor (Hodgkin et al. 1973). It seems that Asian immigrants have a similar vitamin D intake to that of indigenous British people (Stephens et al. 1982) but have much less exposure to sunlight.

Clinical surveys

Hodkinson et al. (1973) investigated 103 consecutive admissions to a geriatric department in North London and considered that the prevalence of osteomalacia lay between 2 and 5% in such persons, being higher in women than in men. A similar study in Glasgow showed a prevalence of 4% in elderly women admitted to hospital (Anderson et al. 1966). Persons admitted to hospital are likely to have been in poorer health than others of their age-group and consequently have had less recent exposure to sunlight. It is therefore not surprising that the prevalence of osteomalacia among old people generally seems to be somewhat lower. Thus the DHSS (1979a) found frank osteomalacia in two out of 365 subjects living at home (0.5%). See Chapter 3 for the role of vitamin D deficiency in fracture of the femur.

Controlled trials

There have been few randomised trials of vitamin D. (See p. 73 for the double-blind trial conducted by Johnson et al. (1980)).

A double-blind trial of factorial design was conducted by Inkovaara et al. (1983) among 327 residents of a home for the elderly. These subjects were randomly allocated to various groups which received all possible combinations of calcium carbonate, vitamin D_3, methandienone and placebo for nine months. The incidence of bone fractures was found to be slightly higher but not significantly higher in groups receiving placebo only. A significant increase occurred in the mortality from coronary disease in groups with any two treatments as compared with less, the increase being greatest for subjects taking vitamin D and methandienone.

Degvun *et al.* (1980) conducted a controlled trial of fluorescent lighting in which one long-stay ward was fitted with lights emitting ultraviolet radiation while another similar ward received ordinary fluorescent light. No significant differences were detected in the patients' plasma 25-HCC concentrations. But in the trial by Corless *et al.* (1978) long-stay patients were randomised individually and received monitored exposure to ultraviolet light, and here a significant rise in plasma 25-HCC occurred.

Comment

Vitamin D deficiency is potentially serious since it causes bone disease. It is especially liable to occur in the housebound, in long-stay patients, and in immigrants, due to insufficient exposure to sunlight. A prevalence of 2–5% for osteomalacia has been reported in old people admitted to hospital, while among the elderly generally it is probably in the order of 0.5%. Subclinical deficiency occurs to an unknown, but probably substantial extent and even if it contributes to a minority of cases of femoral fracture it must be considered an important factor, being in principle preventable.

It is therefore reasonable to enquire what proportion of elderly people would benefit from an increased intake of vitamin D by mouth. This issue is complicated by the possibility that some elderly people are especially sensitive to vitamin D. There is also some evidence of an association between vitamin D and ischaemic heart disease (Dalderup 1973; Knox 1973; Linden 1974), and it is particularly worrying that in a controlled trial coronary mortality should be higher in groups receiving vitamin D. Furthermore, patients with renal stones tend to have a higher vitamin D intake than controls (Taylor 1972). A low vitamin D intake can hardly be termed deficient if the benefits of increasing it may be outweighed by the dangers.

These dangers probably do not apply to skin synthesis of the vitamin. Artificial ultraviolet light can be conveniently supplied in long-stay wards as part of their illumination, but does not seem to affect plasma 25-HCC concentrations. Individual ultraviolet irradiation is effective, but it requires considerable supervision, and the radiation received should preferably be monitored by appropriate badges. If a low vitamin D status is regarded as a deficiency of sunlight, the most logical remedy wherever possible is for the elderly to sit in the sun. It should not be difficult for the hospital authorities to arrange for long-stay patients to enjoy this simple, safe and cheap form of therapy.

FOLIC ACID

The importance of folate deficiency lies in its association with megaloblastic anaemia. Folate absorption and utilisation are affected by certain drugs and alcohol, so that some individuals are at risk of folate deficiency even if their intake is otherwise adequate. Indiscriminate supplementation with folic acid carries the risk of precipitating severe symptoms of vitamin B_{12} deficiency in subjects who have incipient undiagnosed pernicious anaemia.

Intake

The World Health Organisation (1972) group of experts recommended a daily intake of 400 μg for adults. Several studies from different countries suggest that most elderly people receive much less than this amount. MacLeod et al. (1974) found that Glasgow men and women aged 65–74 years had a geometric mean folate intake of 65 μg and 50 μg daily; in subjects aged 75 years and over the daily intakes were 58 μg and 50 μg respectively. In Canadian elderly people, mean daily intakes of 151 μg (men) and 130 μg (women) have been reported, while various groups of elderly people in Florida had mean intakes ranging from 184–250 μg per day (data in Rosenberg et al. 1982). In a Swedish survey elderly men and women were found to have mean folate intakes of 175 and 146 μg per day, respectively (Jagerstad & Westesson 1979). The whole blood folate levels were repeatedly estimated over 6 years and found to be nearly always normal. It has therefore been suggested that the recommended daily intake of 400 μg is too high (Rosenberg *et al.* 1982).

Blood levels

It is usually assumed that a serum folate below 3 ng/ml or a red-cell folate below about 150 ng/ml indicates a high risk of deficiency and by these criteria, many old people seem to be at high risk. The DHSS (1972) survey reported mean serum levels in elderly men and women of 5.8 and 6.4 ng/ml respectively, about 15% falling below 3 ng/ml. Mean red-cell folate values were 250 ng/ml (men) and 253 ng/ml (women), 16% being below 150 ng/ml and 4% below 100 ng/ml, similar results were obtained in a later survey (DHSS 1979a). Elwood *et al.* (1972) reported similar serum folate and somewhat higher red-cell folate levels among elderly English and Welsh subjects. They found that elderly Asian immigrants tended to have a lower folate status than the native-born elderly British. It appears that in Wales folate status is better in elderly women than in younger women (Elwood *et al.* 1971).

Clinical surveys

In several surveys no relationship has been found between folate and haemoglobin concentrations (Elwood *et al.* 1971, 1972; DHSS 1972; Jagerstad & Westesson 1979). The second DHSS (1979a) survey found five cases of folate-deficient anaemia among 365 subjects, plus one person with folate-deficient macrocytosis and a 'low normal' haemoglobin. All these subjects had some chronic illness and most had evidence of other deficiencies. If they represent the general population of old people, the prevalence of folate deficiency is 1–2%. Another 11 subjects (3%) had low folate levels and macrocytosis but no anaemia, and were thought to have subclinical deficiency. Among 51 consecutive persons admitted to an old people's home Read *et al.* (1965) found one case of folate deficiency anaemia, and Batata *et al.* (1967) found no cases of megaloblastic anaemia among 100 elderly patients consecutively admitted to hospital despite many low serum folate values. In this study patients with organic brain disease had significantly lower serum folate levels than those without brain disease. Sneath *et al.* (1973) found an association between a low red-cell folate concentration and dementia in 115 consecutive admissions to a geriatric unit. In contrast, Elwood *et al.* (1971) found no association between folate status and mental function among 533 subjects aged 65 years and over who were living in the community. These findings suggest that impairment of mental function bad enough to warrant admission to hospital, may be associated with poor nutritional state, and that a low folate status is the result, rather than the cause of the intellectual impairment. Alcoholism seems to be particularly associated with 'pure' folate-deficiency megaloblastic anaemia, and so is treatment with anticonvulsants (Rosenberg *et al.* 1982).

Randomised controlled trial

Apart from patients with megaloblastic anaemia (which is uncommon), there is little evidence to suggest that old people need more folic acid than they commonly receive. One controlled trial (unpublished) was conducted by Dr P.C. Elwood among old people living at home in South Wales. Subjects with serum folate levels below 6 ng/ml were randomly allocated to receive folic acid 5 mg daily or matching placebo tablets, together with vitamin B_{12} injections where serum B_{12} was low. After three months a detailed questionnaire on symptoms was administered to 19 subjects receiving folic acid and to 17 subjects receiving placebo, and at the same time a battery of mental-function tests were administered. No significant difference was found between the two groups except that the placebo group reported a greater improvement in general well-being than did the treated group. This difference was presumably fortuitous, but it makes the possibility of real benefit due to folic acid seem unlikely.

Comment

Folic acid deficiency occasionally causes megaloblastic anaemia in the elderly. The prevalence of this condition is probably less than 2% among people over 70 years of age. Folate deficiency cannot be defined solely in terms of intake since the daily requirement is not known, nor is it synonymous with red-cell or serum concentrations below a given value. It is particularly liable to occur (together with other types of malnutrition) in old people who are suffering from chronic illness, dementia or alcoholism.

VITAMIN B_{12}

Deficiency in vitamin B_{12} causes pernicious anaemia and it arises in persons who lack the ability to absorb the vitamin, and in those who usually have a specific abnormality of the gastric mucosa.

Whether subclinical B_{12} deficiency exists is uncertain. Presumably there is a state in the development of pernicious anaemia when it has not yet caused overt anaemia but is detectable biochemically and at any given time some people will be in this phase. The requirements for vitamin B_{12} are very small (3 μg daily) and the vitamin is present in all foods of animal origin so that a simple dietary deficiency is exceedingly rare, but it has occasionally been reported in vegans or others who take a very restricted diet.

Blood concentrations

The serum concentration of vitamin B_{12} is usually above 200 pg/ml, and a value below 100 pg/ml is taken to imply deficiency. In the first DHSS (1972) survey mean values in men and women were 396 and 446 pg/ml, respectively; 1% of subjects had values below 100 pg/ml, and 10% fell in the borderline range of 100-200 pg/ml. Elwood et al. (1972) found somewhat lower mean values, with elderly Asian immigrants having lower concentrations than the indigenous English. With increasing age the mean serum B_{12} concentration declines and a higher proportion of people have low serum levels (Waters et al. 1971; DHSS 1972; Jagerstad et al. 1979). Low serum concentrations occur following partial gastrectomy and in patients with the malabsorption syndrome or atrophic gastritis (which is common in the elderly).

Clinical surveys

The prevalence of pernicious anaemia rises with age owing to the accumulation of persons successfully undergoing treatment with vitamin B_{12}, and it seems to be commoner in women. In a Danish survey the prevalence in men and women aged 70–79 years was 0.5% and 1.1% respectively, while in men and women over the age of 80 years it had risen to 0.9% and 2.4% respectively (Pedersen & Mosbech 1969).

The question arises as to whether any risk to health is implied by a low B_{12} status in the absence of pernicious anaemia. The second DHSS (1979a) survey found several persons who appeared to be generally malnourished and in poor health and also had a low serum B_{12} concentration. Whether the low B_{12} contributed to their ill-health or whether it was merely a reflection of it, was not clear. Cole and Prchal (1984) reported lower serum B_{12} levels in association with Alzheimer-type dementia in the elderly, in comparison with patients suffering from other forms of dementia and with non-demented elderly persons. There was no association between serum B_{12} and the haematological state. The relationship with Alzheimer's disease may have been causal ; it may have arisen from malabsorption or metabolic disturbance consequent upon the disease; it may have been due to an analogue of vitamin B_{12} which interfered with the assay; or it may have been fortuitous. It is obviously desirable that this work should be repeated. Batata *et al.* (1967) found no association between serum B_{12} and the presence of organic brain disease among elderly patients admitted to hospital. Elwood *et al.* (1971) found no association between low serum B_{12} levels and intellectual impairment in a representative sample of 533 subjects over the age of 65 years. Similarly the first DHSS (1972) survey found no significant relationship between serum B_{12} concentration and mental state in 656 elderly subjects.

Prospective study

Serum concentrations of vitamin B_{12} were measured in 673 subjects aged 35–64 years who were followed up for ten years by Waters *et al.* (1971). There was a remarkably high correlation between the results taken from the same subjects ten years apart. Subjects with values below 100 pg/ml on the first occasion were kept under review during the follow-up period, and in eight subjects the serum concentration remained below 100 pg/ml almost continuously without any fall in haemoglobin. There was no association between mortality and low vitamin B_{12} status.

Controlled trial

A further investigation of the potential significance of a low vitamin B_{12} status was undertaken by Hughes *et al.* (1970). A controlled trial was undertaken to test the hypothesis that vitamin B_{12} deficiency, in the absence of macrocytic anaemia or neuropathy, might produce psychiatric symptoms. Thirty-nine subjects over the age of 65 years were found in a survey to have serum B_{12} concentrations below 150 pg/ml, none of them had anaemia or B_{12}-deficient neuropathy, and none were taking drugs likely to interfere with B_{12} metabolism. Half were given intramuscular injections of B_{12} while the others received a placebo injection for five weeks. A detailed assessment of mental state and general well-being was made by a psychiatrist who was unaware of the patients' allocation within the trial. There was no evidence that vitamin B_{12} was superior to placebo in effecting any improvement in the patients' condition, although there was a clear tendency for all the subjects to report an improvement during the trial.

Comment

Vitamin B_{12} deficiency is important because of its association with pernicious anaemia and its neurological sequelae. In view of the potential seriousness of this condition it seems reasonable to suspect low serum B_{12} levels as being prejudicial to health even when they are not accompanied by other evidence of pernicious anaemia but there is little evidence to support this idea. An association between low serum levels and ill-health has been reported in some surveys but not in others; however, since serum B_{12} tends to decline with age, a low value may simply be a marker for biological ageing, particularly of the gastrointestinal tract. The evidence of the prospective study and the controlled trial suggest that a low serum B_{12} is not synonymous with deficiency in the absence of overt pernicious anaemia. A true dietary deficiency of vitamin B_{12} is exceedingly rare in Western communities.

THIAMIN

Classical beriberi is seldom diagnosed in Western society. There is still, however, some concern that lesser degrees of thiamin deficiency may be fairly common in the elderly and contribute to various abnormalities and diseases.

Intake

The various dietary surveys that have been conducted in British elderly people have produced remarkably similar estimates of thiamin intake. The mean amounts taken per day were 0.9–1.1 mg in meₙ and ᴜ.7–0.8 mg in women (DHSS 1972, 1979a; MacLeod et al. 1974; Lonergan et al. 1975). These figures are virtually identical with the daily intakes recommended by the British Department of Health, so that many elderly people have an intake below the recommended level. In relation to total energy intake, however, the thiamin intake of the elderly is equal to that of the general population (DHSS 1972).

Biochemical status

The biochemical method most often used in surveys to assess thiamin status is the TPP effect. Iber et al. (1982) reviewed various surveys and showed wide differences in the proportion who, by their criteria, were thiamin deficient. Thus 68% of geriatric patients admitted to a London hospital (Griffiths et al. 1967) had some degree of biochemical thiamin deficiency (apparently a TPP effect of 15% or more) while none in a survey of elderly residents of Vancouver were thiamin deficient (Leichter et al. 1978). Iber et al. (1982) considered that about 10% of the elderly in the USA had some thiamin deficiency. The DHSS (1972) survey found a TPP effect above 15% in 30 out of 114 subjects (35%), but these people did not have a lower thiamin intake than the others, and neither did those in whom the effect exceeded 23%. This led the DHSS Panel to question whether a high TPP effect necessarily implies thiamin deficiency. In a survey in South Wales, a high TPP effect was associated with living alone in men, but not in women, and with a low ascorbate status in men (Burr et al. 1982).

Clinical surveys

The first DHSS (1972) survey found no association between TPP effect and clinical rating, and the second (DHSS 1979a) found no association with mental test score. In this survey some of the subjects with a low thiamin status seemed to be generally malnourished. Older and Dickerson (1982) reported an association between thiamin deficiency and postoperative confusion. Thiamin deficiency is an important complication of alcoholism, but its prevalence in this connection is unknown. (See Chapter 7).

Prospective study

The study by Kemm and Allcock (1984) examined the prognostic significance of various nutritional indices including erythrocyte transketolase activity. No association was found between this and the mortality of 159 elderly patients.

Controlled trial

Thiamin was included in the multivitamin preparation used in the Farnborough trial (Taylor 1968). A test of myotactic hyper-irritability, thought to reflect thiamin deficiency, was performed every three months on the subjects in the trial. At the end of twelve months there was a substantial and significant difference between the treated and control group in their response to this test. All but 7 of the 80 subjects initially had a low thiamin status.

Comment

It seems that old people take less thiamin than younger persons and may have a lower thiamin status as judged by biochemical tests. It is possible that low thiamin status might contribute to confusion in the elderly. The Farnborough trial suggests that thiamin deficiency may be common in long-stay patients. Further controlled trials are needed to investigate these issues.

RIBOFLAVIN

Deficiency of riboflavin can cause skin lesions, especially around the mouth. These lesions are common in the elderly and it is therefore desirable to know how frequently riboflavin deficiency occurs.

Intake

Four nutritional surveys of elderly British people found mean daily intakes of 1.3–1.7 mg in men and 1.1–1.3 mg in women (DHSS 1972, 1979a; MacLeod et al. 1974; Lonergan et al. 1975). It is therefore clear that a large number of old people have an intake below that officially recommended (1.7 mg for men, 1.3 mg for women).

Biochemical status

Riboflavin status was assessed by means of EGR–AC tests in the DHSS (1979a) survey. Thirty percent of the subjects had EGR–AC values above 1.3, and the proportion was higher in social classes IV and V.

Clinical surveys

Angular stomatitis or cheilosis were found in 57 out of 778 subjects in the DHSS (1972) survey. It was thought that some of these lesions were probably due to riboflavin deficiency, but mean riboflavin intake of this group was almost identical to that of other subjects. The authors considered that it is reasonable to expect a dimunition in riboflavin requirements in old age. In the second DHSS (1979a) survey the clinically malnourished subjects were more likely to have high EGR–AC values than those who appeared to be well nourished.

Prospective study

In the prospective study by Kemm and Allcock (1984) a high EGR–AC value was not found to have any prognostic significance in elderly hospital patients.

Controlled trial

The multivitamin treatment in the Farnborough trial included a daily dose of 15 mg riboflavin. Scars at the angle of the mouth were mainly unaltered by treatment, so that either these lesions were irreversible or they were not caused by riboflavin deficiency.

Comment

Old people in Britain commonly take less riboflavin than is officially recommended, and their biochemical status reflects this. It is possible that riboflavin deficiency makes an important contribution to the mouth and lip lesions commonly found in old people. There is however, little definite evidence available and it seems desirable that randomised trials should be undertaken in persons who have these lesions.

OTHER VITAMINS

Vitamin A intake seems to be adequate in Britain if the recommended intakes are any guide. There is no clinical evidence of deficiency in the elderly. A low retinol status predicted death in the prospective study by Kemm & Allcock (1984), but this is likely to have been a result of the poor condition of patients rather than a cause of it.

Nicotinic acid intakes are usually above recommended levels. About 1% of the subjects in the first DHSS (1972) survey had an inflamed tongue, but it was not specifically attributed to nicotinic acid deficiency. The Farnborough trial included nicotinic acid in its multivitamin preparation, and the assessing physician reported that the earliest sign of improvement occurred in the subjects' tongues, many of which were initially inflamed (Taylor 1968). This trial therefore provides some limited evidence for the existence of nicotinic acid deficiency although it is by no means clear that this was the cause of the glossitis in these patients.

Pyridoxine intake is often below the recommended daily intake level of 2 mg. The four British dietary surveys concur in finding mean intakes of 1.1–1.4 mg in men and 0.8–1.0 in women (DHSS 1972, 1979a; MacLeod et al. 1974; Lonergan et al. 1975). There is no clinical evidence that pyridoxine deficiency occurs in the elderly.

CONCLUSIONS

Many elderly people have a lower intake of vitamins than the levels officially recommended yet it cannot be assumed that such persons are necessarily deficient. It has been found however that many elderly people have a lower vitamin status than is common among younger people. This is especially true for vitamins C and D, for folic acid and in some groups for thiamin. The term 'deficiency' should be reserved for cases where there is clear clinical evidence that vitamin insufficiency has caused some impairment of health or where the subject's biochemical status has been shown to carry a substantial risk of such ill-health.

It is likely that individuals vary in their requirements for several vitamins. It should therefore not be assumed that there is a single optimum intake for all old people. There are dangers attached to a high intake of some vitamins, particularly vitamin D and folic acid, (see Chapter 12) so that the risks of deficiency must be weighed against the risks of excess.

Persons with a low intake or a low vitamin status not infrequently have more evidence of ill health or a greater tendency to die than others of their age-groups. But in most cases the ill-health probably causes the low vitamin status by impairing the patient's appetite or handling of the vitamin, so that it should not be assumed that vitamin deficiency causes the ill health.

Vitamin D deficiency occurs in Britain especially among the housebound, long-stay inpatients and Asian immigrants. The prevalence of frank clinical osteomalacia is about 0.5% in the elderly, but subclinical disease is probably more common. It should be regarded primarily as a deficiency in exposure to sunlight. The prevalence of scurvy is apparently 0.2–0.8% in the elderly; lesser degrees of vitamin C deficiency occur, but their frequency is unknown owing to difficulties of recognition and definition. Old men living alone and long-stay inpatients are most at risk.

Folic acid deficiency causes megaloblastic anaemia in 1–2% of the elderly. The prevalence of thiamin, riboflavin and other B vitamin deficiencies in the elderly is unknown.

6   Water Soluble Vitamins, Neuro-transmitters and Brain Biochemistry

J. Greenwood, O.E. Pratt, G.K. Shaw &
A.D. Thomson

CLASSIFICATION OF MINOR NUTRIENTS

B group vitamins, essential amino acids and trace metals share many physiological characteristics and it is largely due to historical accident that they have come to be treated separately. The usual definition of vitamins as organic substances required in trace amounts for normal growth and health poses some difficulties in classification. Thus choline may be needed in the diet because it can only be synthesised in the body from other essential nutrients, but choline is not usually regarded as a vitamin. Retinol and the amino acid tryptophan are both needed by humans in quantities of 5–10 μg/Kg body weight daily, but by custom only the former is classified as a vitamin. Similarly both trace metals and B group vitamins are required in quantities of a few mg or μg and share the role of being co-factors for enzymes.

Some 50 years ago Rose and his collaborators distinguished between the 8 or 10 essential amino acids which must be present in mammalian diet and the non-essential amino acids which could be synthesised. This important distinction has to be modified when considering the nutritional needs of the brain since not all of the so called non-essential amino acids can be synthesised by brain cells (Table 6.1). Tyrosine for example can readily be made from phenylalanine in liver cells but not in brain cells and therefore has to be included among the organ-essential amino acids which must reach the brain from the blood to ensure its adequate nutrition. Choline is another nutrient which can be made in the liver (from the essential amino acid methionine) but not in the brain which must obtain either choline or choline containing phospholipids from the blood.

Table 6.1   The 'organ essential' nutrients which the
brain needs for its proper metabolism and function,
but cannot synthesise for itself although they may be
synthesised elsewhere in the body.

The generally accepted vitamins
'Essential' amino acids
'Essential' fatty acids
Inorganic trace elements

Other amino acids
  Tyrosine, Serine, Histidine, Arginine, Citrulline

Many nucleotides and nucleic acid precursors

Hormones
  Triiodothyronine, Adrenocortical steroids

Miscellaneous
  e.g., peptides such as carnitine

The category of organ essential nutrients includes many
nucleic acid precursors (Cornford & Oldendorf 1975) and thyroid
hormones which are required by all tissues. Thyroid hormones
can fairly readily cross the blood–brain barrier (Pratt 1981).
Examples of organ essential minor nutrients needed by the brain
are summarised in Table 6.1. Any interference in later life with
the supply of these nutrients to the brain will almost certainly be
harmful.

THE INTERFACE BETWEEN THE BRAIN AND BLOOD

Various dyes when injected intravenously stain other tissues but
not the brain and disturbances in blood electrolytes affect the
brain much later than they affect other tissues such as the heart.
The basis of this protection is the special nature of the blood
capillaries of the brain. Unlike most other capillaries, they
have a tight junction between the cells so that their surface
membranes form a barrier, commonly known as the blood–brain
barrier. The only molecules which can cross this barrier and
enter the brain are: (1) a few very small or lipid soluble molecules
and (2) those which have a special transport mechanism. Most

water-soluble nutrients cross the barrier by specific carrier-mediated transport mechanisms, which like enzymes can be saturated by high concentrations of the substrate and competitively inhibited by chemical analogues of the substrate. For most nutrients there is also a small non-saturable component which is likely to be passive diffusion (Figure 6.1).

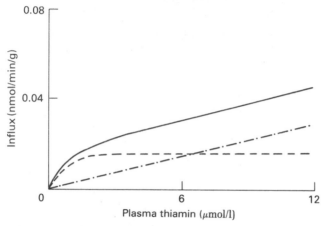

Fig. 6.1   The components of thiamin transport across the blood–brain barrier, the saturable component (- - -), the apparently non-saturable component (-·-·-), the sum of the two components (——) (based on data of Greenwood & Pratt 1983). Note that normally blood plasma thiamin concentration is well below 1 μmol/l so that the flux is mainly due to the saturable component. If the thiamin level is raised, the proportion due to the non-saturable component increases becoming the major contribution as the concentration exceeds 6 μmol/l.

Although the non-saturable component accounts for less than 10% of the transport across the blood–brain barrier in normal physiological conditions, it may become very important if the saturable carrier-mediated process is severely inhibited or defective for any reason. In these circumstances if blood levels of a nutrient can be raised sufficiently high by therapeutic doses of that nutrient (for example B vitamins) it can be forced across the blood–brain barrier using the non-saturable non-inhibitable component.

The effect of age upon the blood–brain barrier transport systems

There is evidence that the properties of many carrier-mediated transport systems for nutrients in the blood–brain barrier change with age. The monocarboxylic acid transport system in the blood–brain barrier of the rat is almost inactive at birth but rapidly increases to a high capacity in early life and then declines again in the adult (Cremer *et al.* 1976; Daniel *et al.* 1977). The system is important as it enables ketone bodies, produced by lipid metabolism, to replace glucose as energy source for the brain during ketoacidosis produced by fasting or by the high fat diet of suckling. Neutral amino acids enter the brain in the suckling rat at a greater rate than in the adult. This indicates a greater activity of the suckling rat's transport systems, although the higher levels of these amino acids in the circulation also contribute to the higher rate of influx (Banos *et al.* 1978; Daniel *et al.* 1978). On the other hand transport of glucose across the blood–brain barrier is low in young rats and only rises to adult levels as the rats mature (Daniel *et al.* 1978).

There is some evidence that the transport of both glucose and amino acids across the blood–brain barrier declines in late adulthood. Glucose transport in elderly rats (64 weeks old) was reduced to 0.57 ± 0.02 (mean ± SE) from 0.97 ± 0.09 μmol/min/g brain in young adults (Daniel *et al.* 1978). Thiamin transport across the gut wall is reduced in old rats (Lazarov 1977) but not in humans (Thomson 1966), or across the blood–brain barrier of the rat. In thirteen rats more than 20 months old the thiamin flux into the brain was 0.0284 + 0.0030 compared with 0.0271 ± 0.0021 μmol/min/g brain in 78 young adult rats (Greenwood & Pratt unpublished).

It is not clear whether any possible impairment of transport in later life is due to a reduction in the number of carrier molecules, to a reduced effectiveness of existing carriers, or through loss of affinity for the substance being transported (Daniel *et al.* 1978). Pathological deterioration of the cell surfaces and accumulation of transcription errors in the synthesis of special carrier proteins, and many other changes may all contribute to a reduction in transport rates.

Competitive inhibition of blood–brain barrier transport systems

One possible cause of trouble is inhibition of the specific transport carriers in the cell walls of the cerebral blood capillaries. Such inhibition is most likely to be due to competition for the carrier between substances with similar chemical structures. Kinetic analysis shows that competition between amino acids for shared transport carriers in the blood–brain barrier is usually so severe that the rate of flux across the barrier is no more than a small fraction of what it would be if no other amino acid were present in the blood plasma (Banos, Daniel & Pratt 1971; 1974; Pratt 1976; 1979; 1980b; 1982). This competition is important for it means that an abnormality in the pattern of amino acids relative to one another in the blood may interfere with the supply of one or more limiting amino acids to the brain. This mechanism is likely to play a part in malnutrition and in other possible metabolic disturbance in old age.

B vitamins tend to have dissimilar structures and do not compete with each other for transport. However transport of B vitamins across the blood–brain barrier may be inhibited by chemical analogues as in the case of thiamin (Greenwood & Pratt 1983). Such analogues generally do not occur naturally though one is widely used in animal husbandry and others may be formed by the action of microorganisms on thiamin in the gut.

DEFICIENCY STATES AND CENTRAL NEUROTRANSMITTERS

Lack of almost any of the B group vitamins if sufficiently severe leads to some neuropsychiatric disturbance. The mechanism by which the deficiency affects the central nervous system is usually not clear but often involves disturbances of amino acid metabolism. Pellagra furnishes one example of the many close links between deficiencies of B group vitamins and amino acid metabolism. The disease is due to niacin deficiency but develops only if the diet is also deficient in tryptophan since otherwise the vitamin can be synthesised from this essential amino acid.

CHRONIC ALCOHOLISM

Chronic alcoholism is commonly associated with nutritional deficiency in later life. The very same factors of loneliness and deteriorating mental function which predispose to alcoholism are also likely to increase the risk of secondary malnutrition. Since the mechanism of alcohol addiction is widely believed to be rooted in neurotransmitter function it is possible that nutritional deficiencies especially of thiamin or essential amino acids may aggravate any neurotransmitter disturbance and lead to a vicious spiral of deterioration. More research is needed in this important field.

ACQUIRED AND INHERITED METABOLIC OR TRANSPORT DEFECTS

A large number of metabolic errors of amino acid metabolism have been described. Many of these lead to abnormal accumulation of one or more amino acids in the circulation which may competitively inhibit transport systems and impair the supply of organ essential amino acids to the central nervous system. One well known example of such a disorder is phenylketonuria in which there is an accumulation of phenylalanine which may competitively inhibit transport across the blood–brain barrier and possibly lead to lack of methionine, tryptophan and other amino acids (Pratt 1980a). The effects of such genetically determined defects usually appear early in life, but are sometimes delayed until adult life. If the effect were delayed into old age its genetic basis would be difficult to establish but this might be the basis of some types of presenile dementia. Another possibility is that the genetic defect does not of itself lead directly to an overt metabolic error but predisposes to further damage as in the 'fragile X' syndrome in which the X chromosome is unduly susceptible to damage during cell division. There are other conditions in which the enzyme deficiency is partial rather than total and the defect may not become apparent until other disorders in later life impose a greater load upon the metabolism. In one such disorder, cystathione synthetase deficiency, many patients can be helped by being given large doses of vitamin B_6, the co-factor for the affected enzyme to produce maximum possible activity and relatively normal metabolic function (Mudd & Levy 1978). In old age, there may be some slight impairment of vitamin B_6 absorption from the gastrointestinal tract. This would not affect a normal person but may exacerbate problems in recognised cases of cystathione synthetase deficiency and produce symptoms for the first time in undiagnosed less severe cases. It seems likely that careful, combined nutritional and metabolic study in old age will reveal conditions due to partial deficiency of some of the many vitamin dependent enzymes which are only revealed when the nutrient supply is marginal.

METABOLIC EFFECTS OF DEFICIENCY OF MINOR NUTRIENTS IN OLD AGE

The effects of deficiency of minor nutrients such as B group vitamins in the elderly are similar to those in younger people. Chronic mild deficiency of B group vitamins is difficult to diagnose in the elderly because of the prevalence of other causes of similar syndromes and minor neuropsychiatric problems. The vitamin dependent enzymes are interesting not only because they indicate possible mechanisms by which central nervous system damage might be caused, but also because (see Chapter 4) they provide sensitive indicators of mild degrees of vitamin deficiency (Dreyfus 1962; Blass & Gibson 1977; Greenwood et al. 1984).

It is important to consider not only the blood levels of B group vitamins and similar micronutrients but also the adequacy of their supply to the brain. It must be remembered that all water soluble vitamins are polar and will only be able to cross the blood–brain barrier or choroid plexus to any extent with the help of a carrier-mediated transport system (Spector 1982). Carrier-mediated transport has been described for many substances in this class including vitamin C (Chatamra et al. 1985), choline (Cornford et al. 1978) and complex substances like B_{12} (Bhatt et al. 1980). Most work, however, has been done on thiamin transport which will be discussed here as an illustrative example.

Transport of thiamin across the blood–brain barrier

The rate of influx of thiamin provided by the non-saturable component of flux within the normal plasma range is not sufficient to meet the needs of the brain (Greenwood *et al*, 1982; Reggiani *et al*. 1984) and the carrier mechanism is therefore vital for normal cerebral function. Moreover the rate of total thiamin influx is of the same order of magnitude as turnover. This implies that when circulating thiamin levels are low, influx may be insufficient to meet cellular requirements (Rindi *et al*. 1980; Greenwood *et al*. 1982). Thiamin deficiency with a reduced level of the vitamin in the blood may occur in the elderly who have a poor diet and impaired intestinal absorption of the vitamin. This is particularly likely in the malnourished chronic alcoholic patient (Thomson *et al*. 1970). The thiamin reserves in tissue are small and easily depleted by losses of thiamin in perspiration and urine (Pearson 1967) and urinary losses cannot be reduced as there is no renal tubular reabsorption of thiamin (Carleen *et al*. 1944). Raising blood thiamin concentrations can raise its flux into the brain by both the carrier-mediated and non-saturable components of transport (Figure 6.1). This may be relevant to the nutritional treatment of various conditions including chronic alcoholism (Pratt 1980b; Thomson 1982; Greenwood & Pratt 1984) and Leigh's disease (Pincus *et al*. 1971; Pincus *et al*. 1976).

There is a disease of ruminants known as cerebrocortical necrosis which responds to adequate dosage of thiamin (Edwin & Jackman 1973). Thiamin analogues produced in the gut by micro-organisms play a part in the pathogenesis of this condition, and the neuropsychiatric signs that the central nervous system is being deprived of thiamin may occur while the circulating levels of thiamin remain within normal limits. Similar conditions have not yet been reported in man but when there is any severe disturbance of gastrointestinal function there is a possibility that analogues of the B group vitamins may be produced within the gut by micro-organisms. Normal blood thiamin levels would all too easily divert attention from the possibility of an inadequate vitamin supply to the brain as a cause of the clinical manifestation.

Whatever the reason, a thiamin deficiency state in the elderly is dangerous in view of the possible reduction in blood–brain barrier transport of the vitamin with ageing. The deficiency can be treated by raising the blood concentration of thiamin to a level sufficiently high to overcome competitive inhibition and increase the influx by the non-saturable process. An alternative may be to give lipid-soluble derivatives of thiamin which are not restricted from entering the central nervous system, but release free thiamin into the metabolic pool after crossing the blood–brain barrier as the lipid soluble moiety is split off enzymatically in the brain cells (Pincus et al. 1971; Thomson et al. 1971).

Sir Archibald Garrod first propounded the concept of inborn predisposition in relation to enzymes but it seems just as likely to apply to transport processes. Carrier molecules behave in many respects like enzymes and within any population the values of Jmax, the maximum flux with excess of substrate and Kt the affinity constant of the carrier for its substrate for transport into the brain will vary due to chemical individuality (Garrod 1931; Childs & Der Kaloustian 1968; Childs 1970). Due to this variability certain individuals may possess sufficient carrier activity to provide an adequate supply of water soluble nutrients into the brain under normal conditions, but not sufficient during a period of biochemical stress such as alcoholism or a degenerative process associated with old age.

It has been suggested that thiamin deficiency itself can cause a breakdown of the blood–brain barrier (Warnock & Burkhalter 1968) but it seems that this does not occur until there is tissue necrosis and haemorrhage (Robertson & Manz 1971; Manz & Robertson 1972). We have used tracer labelled mannitol, a substance for which there is no carrier-mediated transport system to measure the integrity of the blood–brain barrier. Normally this substance crosses the barrier at a slow rate with an apparent transfer constant less than 1 μl/min/g brain tissue (Daniel et al. 1981; Deane et al. 1984). In the thiamin deficient rat cerebrum the apparent transfer constant was 0.82 $\pm$ 0.13 μl/min/g brain tissue (mean + SE of 4 estimates) and not significantly different from the value of 0.76 $\pm$ 0.09 μl/min/g (mean $\pm$ SE of 6 estimates) in a control group (Greenwood & Pratt unpublished).

Defects of carrier processes within animals are difficult to demonstrate but a mutant strain of Escherichia coli that possesses a defective thiamin transport system and requires a thiamin concentration in the growth medium 150 fold higher than the parent strain, has been isolated (Kawasaki *et al.* 1969). In mammals the effect of a defect in a transport carrier for a vitamin or similar nutrient could range from being fatal shortly after conception to being subclinical under normal conditions. There have been reports of malabsorption syndromes in which the carriers for folic acid and vitamin B$_{12}$ transport are defective (Lanzkowsky *et al.* 1969; Corcino *et al.* 1970). More recently there have been reports of abnormally low cerebrospinal fluid folate levels with reduced CSF/plasma ratios in the Kearns-Sayre syndrome (Allan *et al.* 1983; Dougados *et al.* 1983) a finding consistent with a possible defect of folate transport across the blood–brain barrier in these patients. It is possible that defects of transport systems, especially intestinal ones, may be acquired as part of the metabolic disturbances suffered in old age.

The maintenance of relatively constant levels of thiamin within the brain during a state of deficiency when other organs rapidly lose thiamin might be the result of thiamin binding more tightly to its dependent enzymes in the central nervous system than in other tissues. However the turnover of thiamin within the central nervous system in rats is from 2–10% of the total thiamin content per hour which is similar in order of magnitude to the turnover in other tissues (Rindi *et al.* 1980; Sen & Cooper 1976). The affinity of thiamin dependent enzymes in the brain does not appear to be different from that in other tissues (Blass *et al.* 1982). Loss of thiamin from the brain is mainly due to net efflux of free thiamin by carrier facilitated diffusion at the capillary endothelium. The rate of this efflux will only become critical when blood and capillary thiamin levels drop sufficiently to establish a concentration gradient conducive to efflux.

It can be concluded that the movement of thiamin into the central nervous system is restricted by both the blood–brain barrier and the limitations of the carrier process. Adequate supplies of the vitamin to the brain can only be achieved when the concentration of free thiamin in the blood plasma is sufficiently greater than that in the brain extracellular space. The efflux of free thiamin from the brain to the blood also appears to be limited and is likely to be further reduced in old age. These phenomena protect the central nervous system during adverse conditions by maintaining near normal levels of thiamin within the brain for long periods.

Minor nutrients, Amino acid metabolism and brain function

The close dependence of central neurotransmitters upon the availability and metabolism of amino acids points to the importance of the supply to the organ not only of the amino acids which it needs but also of other minor trace nutrients including B group vitamins and trace metals which are co-factors for many of the enzymes of amino acid metabolism. Many individual amino acids including some of the non-essential ones have important roles in the metabolism and function of the central nervous system (Table 6.2).

Table 6.2   Some of the more important thiamin dependant enzymes.

Pyruvate dehydrogenase complex
    Converts pyruvic acid to acetyl co-enzyme A. This is a link between glycolysis and the tricarboxylic acid cycle.

Transketolase
    Converts e.g. pentose sugars xylulose phosphate and ribose phosphate to a mixture of the heptose sugar sedoheptulose and the common triose glyceraldehyde.

α-Ketoacid decarboxylase
    Acts on the α-ketoacids formed from the branched chain amino acids, isoleucine, leucine and valine.

α-Ketoglutarate dehydrogenase complex
    A key enzyme for the regulation of the energy yielding tricarboxylic acid cycle.

(Many other thiamin dependant enzymes have been described, but have not yet been found in the mammalian brain.)

Most neurotransmitters established, putative or probable, are either amino acids, (e.g. glutamate or glycine) or formed directly from amino acids, (e.g. catechol amines) or dependent upon the availability of amino acids for their synthesis, (e.g.

acetylcholine). It is important to remember that almost all amino acids which cross the blood–brain barrier are used to repair or replace protein much of which passes down the processes of nerve cells to be used at cell surfaces in ways which are not fully understood. However even though the usage of amino acids in central neurotransmitter synthesis is quantitatively unimportant (except where the neurotransmitter is itself an amino acid) any abnormality in the pattern of free amino acids in the tissue which may occur in old age will be likely to affect neurotransmitter synthesis. Any imbalance in the pattern of free amino acids is likely to be aggravated by the removal of most of the available amino acids in fixed proportions for protein synthesis. A lack of any particular amino acid is likely to have important effects upon the direction and balance of neurotransmitter synthesis as indicated by the relations shown in Table 6.2.

Butterworth (1982) has reviewed the evidence that neurotransmitter function is disturbed in thiamin deficiency. He suggests that the deficiency primarily leads to a central muscarinic cholinergic lesion which partly explains the neurologic deficits in this condition. A decrease in the activity of the thiamin pyrophosphate dependent pyruvate dehydrogenase complex could interfere with acetylcholine synthesis (Table 6.3) and the selective vulnerability of different brain structures to thiamin lack could be related to their normal thiamin turnover rate. There is a striking increase in turnover of serotonin in the hippocampus and hypothalamus of severely thiamin deficient rats (Plaitakis et al. 1982) as well as a number of other changes in central neurotransmitter metabolism. When assessing the relation between thiamin deficiency and neurotransmitter disturbance it is difficult to establish whether these disturbances are the cause or the result of the neurological deficit.

One way in which amino acid metabolism and neurotransmitters are related can be illustrated by the disorder Parkinsonism which is common in later life. The progressive neurological disability associated with this condition appears to be the result of a degenerative process specifically affecting the cells producing the neurotransmitter dopamine. To a certain extent the condition is amenable to treatment with the precursor amino acid L-dihydroxyphenylalanine from which the neurotransmitter is made. The brain cells normally make this pre-

Table 6.3 Some relations between neurotransmitter function and the supply and metabolism of vitamins and other essential minor nutrients.

Neurotransmitter	Particular nutrient requirements of brain
Acetylcholine	Choline or methionine to supply the methyl groups
Catecholamines	The amino acid tyrosine
Dopamine	Either tyrosine or its derivative dihydroxyphenylalanine (Levadopa)
Serotonin	The amino acid tryptophan
Glutamate	Regulation and removal through amino acid metabolism must be important but is poorly understood
All amino acid derived transmitters	Pyridoxine group of vitamins provide co-factors for many steps in metabolism

cursor from tyrosine rather than obtain it from the blood but fortunately L-dihydroxyphenylalanine is readily transported across the blood–brain barrier (Pratt 1976) unlike dopamine which does not easily cross the barrier. There is a possibility that newly devised ways of releasing the missing neurotransmitter at a steady rate within the central nervous system might lead to improved treatment of this condition (Bodor & Simpkins 1983).

An imbalance in the production of one or more of the central neurotransmitters is one possible cause of psychiatric disorder such as depression or neurological disorder such as tremor in old age. For example a relative lack of dopamine might be expected to produce symptoms similar to Parkinsonism but without progressive deterioration. Such a condition is likely to escape diagnosis in view of the difficulty of monitoring nutrient supply to the central nervous system or amino acid levels within brain cells although some sort of indication might be provided by any abnormal amino acid pattern in the CSF.

NUTRITIONAL DEFICIENCY AND BRAIN DAMAGE IN LATER LIFE

Recent technical developments are making it possible to monitor more accurately the insidious development of the sort of damage which may occur through nutritional deficiency in later life using a combination of computerised axial tomography and psychometric testing. Because it develops cumulatively even extensive damage often passes clinically unnoticed in the elderly. Marginal deficiencies of the vitamins and especially of thiamin, nicotinic acid, pyridoxal and vitamin B_{12} may produce alterations in behaviour while more severe deficiencies may produce irreversible changes in cerebral structure. Structural brain changes especially in the midbrain region can be found at post-mortem in patients with thiamin deficiency who are alcoholic and develop the classical Wernicke-Korsakoff syndrome (Victor *et al.* 1971) with drowsiness, confusion, ataxia, abnormal occular movements and an amnesic confabulatory state. However the post-mortem changes are found much more commonly than the condition is diagnosed in life which suggests that the milder forms of the condition often go unrecognised. These milder forms are likely to be characterised by changes in affect and considered judgement, associated with impaired memory, conditions which are commonly found in the elderly for a variety of causes. Another vitamin deficiency likely to cause trouble in the elderly is lack of nicotinic acid (combined with a low tryptophan intake) which causes pellagra with diffuse lesions in the cerebral cortex, basal ganglia, floor of the fourth ventricle and cerebellum. In less severe degrees of this deficiency, behavioural disturbances are likely. Deficiency of the pyridoxal vitamins can also produce both electrophysiological and behavioural changes of varying severity.

In conclusion the primary aim of therapy must be to identify deficiency states at as early a stage as possible so as to be able to prevent the progression towards irreversible structural brain damage. Any predisposing or aggravating factors such as hidden alcohol abuse or malabsorption must also be detected and treated. If deterioration in blood–brain carrier mechanisms proves to be part and parcel of the ageing process it will be an indication that the elderly need higher blood nutrient levels than younger adults. The older the patient the greater is the likelihood that improved nutrition and vitamin supplementation are required.

7 Infections, Vitamins and Confusion in the Elderly

J.H. Puxty

INTRODUCTION

Illness in the elderly provides a considerable diagnostic challenge because it so often presents without the classical symptoms and signs of disease generally seen in the pre-retirement population. Infections of various types are common in this group (Phair 1979) but are frequently not diagnosed as they generally present with problems such as confusion, incontinence, immobility and falling rather than the more classical symptoms of productive cough, dyspnoea and pyrexia. The commonest cause of death in the elderly remains bronchopneumonia and post-mortem evidence suggests that a number of pneumonic illnesses are undiagnosed and untreated during life (Puxty et al. 1983).

Age related changes within the immune mechanisms recently reviewed by Fox (1984) could contribute to the atypical presentations of infection in the elderly. Some changes such as thymic involution and dysfunction of suppressor T cell lines seem virtually universal although there may be some individual variation possibly as a result of differences in the HLA antigens. Other observations such as anergy (Roberts-Thompson et al. 1974), impaired humoral response to vaccines (Phair et al. 1978) and presence of autoantibodies (Hooper et al. 1972) appear to be due to age related disease processes rather than ageing itself and are negative markers of longevity. A variety of modifiers of immune function are recognised including sepsis (Phair 1979; Puxty & Fox 1984a), antibiotics (Eickenberg et al. 1982), hormones (Fabris et al. 1972), changes in carbohydrate tolerance (Puxty & Fox 1984b) and nutrition (Chandra & Newberne 1977).

Malnutrition is known to have profound effects upon the

immune system (Table 7.1). Clinicians have long observed that undernutrition predisposes the host to acquired infections and increases the severity and mortality of infectious illnesses and the likelihood of complications. Infection in turn frequently worsens the nutritional status and may precipitate overt symptoms and signs of malnutrition. A variety of pathogenetic mechanisms probably underlie these interactions (Figure 7.1).

Table 7.1   Effect of protein-energy malnutrition on immune function.

Function	Effect

Lymphoid Tissue
    T Cells
	Atrophy
	Numbers reduced
	Mitogen proliferation to
	    Phytohaemagglutinin A reduced

Delayed hypersensitivity B Cells	Primary and secondary depressed Numbers normal Normal mitogen response to pokeweed
Immunoglobulins	Serum IgA and IgE usually elevated Secretary IgA depressed
Complement	Levels depressed Circulating immune reflexes in 30% Opsonic function of plasma reduced
Phagocytes	Migration impaired Reduced *in vivo* phagocytosis Metabolism and antimicrobial activity reduced

This chapter examines the evidence concerning the interactions of infection and nutrition with reference to vitamins. As isolated deficiencies are rare in clinical practice information from animal studies forms the bulk of the available data. These interactions may possibly explain some of the changes in host defence responses to infection observed in the elderly.

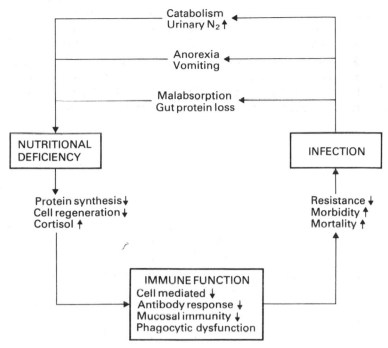

Fig. 7.1   Mechanisms of interactions between infection and nutrition.

EFFECT OF VITAMIN STATUS ON THE RESPONSE TO INFECTION AND THE IMMUNE SYSTEM

Vitamin A

The interactions of vitamin A and the immune system summarised in Table 7.2 have been reviewed by Olson (1972) and Darip *et al.* (1979). Vitamin A has a vital role in maintaining the integrity of epithelial tissue surfaces (Guggenheim & Buechler 1947) which are important, particularly in the respiratory tract for resisting infection. Vitamin A is also required for the production of lacrimal salivary and sweat gland lysosomes.

Table 7.2   Effects of vitamin A deficiency on immune function.

Function	Effect
Lymphoid tissue	Atrophic
Lymphocyte count	May be increased
Antibody response to immunisation	May be suppressed
Lymphocyte transformation	Mitogen response may be decreased
Delayed hypersensitivity	May be suppressed
Peritoneal macrophages	Mobilisation may be reduced

Animal studies (Wissler 1947; Newberne et al. 1968; Bang et al. 1972) suggest a role of vitamin A in the maintenance of lymphocyte and plasma cell populations in the upper respiratory tract. Viral infections (Weather 1946; Panda et al. 1964) are more severe in vitamin A deficient animals. Vitamin A deficient rats are more susceptible to Trypanosome infections and to bacterial infections than are pair fed controls (Jaeger & Muller 1963). Vitamin A deficient dogs exposed to Toxocara develop heavier infestations than controls fed on an adequate diet (Wright 1935).

Vitamins D & E

Increased susceptibility to experimental salmonella infections has been observed in vitamin D deficient rats (Robertson & Ross 1932; McClung & Winter 1932) and in vitamin D deficient piglets (Manniger 1928).

Hamilton et al. (1977) demonstrated impaired peritoneal inflammatory response in Vitamin E deficient rabbits. Vitamin E supplementation has beneficial effects on humoral immunity (Barber et al. 1977; Harman et al. 1977; Heinzerling et al. 1974; Campbell et al. 1974), phagocytic function (Heinzerling et al. 1974) and T cell function (Campbell et al. 1974; Corwin & Schloss 1980). There appears to be a synergism between the immuno-stimulatory effects of vitamin E and other antioxidants particularly selenium (Heinzerling *et al.* 1974; Dreizan 1979). However megadose quantities of vitamin E were shown to reduce *in vitro* neutrophil bactericidal activity and lymphocyte response to Phytohaemagglutinin A (Prasad 1980).

The acid fast bacillae of human leprosy will not normally grow in the hamster and rat, but it will grow if they are made vitamin E deficient (Mason & Bergel 1955). Vitamin E supplementation increases resistance of chickens to *Escherichia Coli* infection (Heinzerling *et al.* 1974).

Vitamin C

The interaction of vitamin C with host defence mechanisms has probably attracted more interest than that of any other vitamin (Table 7.3).

Table 7.3 Effects of vitamin C deficiency on immune function.

Function	Effect
Lymphocyte count	T cell percentage may fall
Allograft survival	Prolonged
Delayed hypersensitivity	Recall mechanisms suppressed
Neutrophil chemotaxis	Mobilisation and *in vitro* motility impaired
Neutrophil metabolism	May be reduced
Macrophages	Mobilisation impaired Size and mobility reduced Fragility increased

Cameron and Pauling (1974) suggested that cell mediated immunity was impaired by vitamin C deficiency. Deficiency may reduce phagocytic cell function (Goetzl *et al.* 1974; Smith *et al.* 1975; Shilotri 1977a; 1977b) and affect the local inflammatory response leading to reduced and delayed cutaneous hypersensitivity reactions (Zweiman *et al.* 1966). Laboratory studies show scorbutic animals to be more susceptible to bacterial, rickettsial and protozoal infections (Scrimshaw, *et al.* 1968).

Folic acid & vitamin B$_{12}$

There is some evidence for impaired humoral responses in folic acid deficiency (Wertmann *et al.* 1952) and the proliferative response of lymphocytes to mitogens may be impaired (Gross *et al.* 1975; Gross & Newberne 1980). Dogs deprived of folic acid after weaning have reduced resistance to infection with *Salmonella typhimurium* (Williams *et al.* 1972).

There have been relatively few studies on the immunological effects of vitamin B$_{12}$. Patients with pernicious anaemia show a decreased ability to phagocytose and kill *Staphylococcus aureus* and to initiate hexose monophosphate shunt activity during phagocyte activation (Kaplan & Basford 1976). A reduced lymphocytic response to Phytohaemagglutinin A has also been reported (MacCuish *et al.* 1974). Vitamin B$_{12}$ supplementation of rats during pregnancy and lactation conferred on their progeny an increased resistance to *Salmonella typhimurium* infection (Newberne & Gebhardt 1973).

Other water soluble vitamins

Pyridoxine deficiencies profoundly effect immune function as summarised in Table 7.4 (Axelrod & Trakatellis 1964; Beisel *et al.* 1981) and depress both humoral (Pruzansky & Axelrod 1955; Hodges *et al.* 1962b) and cell mediated immunity (Fisher *et al.* 1958; Axelrod *et al.* 1963; Robson & Schwarz 1975a; 1975b; Dobbelstein 1974). No consistent interaction has been observed between pyridoxine deficiency and infectious disease (Scrimshaw *et al.* 1968) but pyridoxine deficient rat litters have a higher mortality from bacterial infections (Robson & Schwartz 1975b).

Pantothenic acid deficiencies produce a depression of humoral immune function (Axelrod *et al.* 1947; Hodges *et al.* 1962a) but not of cell mediated immunity. In laboratory animals pantothenic acid deficiency is associated with increased resistance to systemic viral and protozoal infections and decreased resistance to most others (Scrimshaw *et al.* 1968).

Table 7.4   Effects of pyridoxine deficiency on immune function.

Function	Effect
Lymphoid tissue	Atrophic
Lymphocyte count	Depressed
Antibody response to Immunisation*	Primary and Secondary depressed
In *vitro* lymphocyte responses	Diminished in mixed cultures
Delayed hypersensitivity	Depressed
Allograft survival	Prolonged
Neutrophil function	May be diminished

* (Antibody response to immunisation may also be depressed in deficiencies of pantothenic acid, riboflavin, biotin and thiamin)

Riboflavin deficiency similarly results in diminished ability to generate humoral antibodies (Pruzansky & Axelrod 1955) and decreases resistance to most infections (Scrimshaw et al. 1968).

Thiamin deficiencies do not impair the immune system but do increase susceptibility to many bacterial infections (Scrimshaw et al. 1968).

NUTRITIONAL CONSEQUENCES OF INFECTION

Infectious disease is associated with loss of body constituents, rapid utilisation of body nutrient stores and redistribution between various physiological compartments (Table 7.5). The propensity of infections to provoke overt clinical signs of avitaminosis suggests that the septic process has an important effect on vitamin nutriture, however, surprisingly little is known of vitamin metabolism in infection (Vitale 1977).

Vitamin A

In children, concentrations of vitamin A in the blood are appreciably reduced in pneumonia, tonsillitis and rheumatic fever. There are a number of references to vitamin A deficiency pre-

Table 7.5   Possible nutritional consequences of infection.

Absolute Losses
   Increased urinary nitrogen
   Loss of electrolytes, minerals and proteins with vomiting and
      diarrhoea
   Proteinuria
   Negative metabolic balance of minerals, cations and trace
      elements

Functional wastage
   Overutilisation
      Increase usage of metabolic substrates
      Depletion of glycogen stores
      Diversion of amino acids for gluconeogenesis
      Fat mobilisation
      Increased synthesis of cholesterol and triglycerides

Diversion
      Hepatic uptake of nutrients
      Synthesis of acute phase proteins
      Increased hepatocyte synthesis of enzymes

Sequestration
      Uptake of mineral (Fe, Zn) into liver parenchymal cells
      Uptake of trace elements into liver and other organs

---

cipitated by superimposed infections (Scrimshaw *et al.* 1968) but
there have been few controlled studies in either man or animals.
Rats, on a marginally deficient diet, develop overt signs of
vitamin A deficiency when they were infected unless they were
given vitamin A supplements (Newberne *et al.* 1968).

Vitamin C

As early as 1917 Hess drew attention to the frequency with
which children from low socio-economic groups developed florid
scurvy after contracting a febrile illness. Infections produce a
marked depression in plasma and buffy layer ascorbic acid
levels, these findings, however, require cautious interpretation.
Values will alter with changes in leucocyte count (Vallance 1978)
proportions of granulocytes, monocytes, platelets and erythrocytes (Evans *et al.* 1982), season (Andrews *et al.* 1966), age (Loh &

Wilson 1971) and nutrition. It is possible that the changes seen in infection relate to the leucocytosis and represent a change in compartmentalisation rather than a real depletion of body stores (Vitale 1977).

Pauling (1970) popularised the idea that megadose quantities of vitamin C (> 1 g/day) increased resistance to upper respiratory tract infections. There have been several large trials of the efficacy of vitamin C in preventing colds in children and young adults (Anderson *et al.* 1975; Chalmers 1975; Tyrell *et al.* 1977). The interpretation of the results of these trials is disputed but most conclude that vitamin C supplements confer little or no protection though there may be some modest reduction of symptom severity (Baird *et al.* 1979). The benefit of megadose vitamin C in preventing infection in the elderly or any other age group remains unproven.

Thiamin

A number of animal experiments suggest that thiamin status alters with infection (Scrimshaw *et al.* 1968). Anecdotal reports during the second World War suggest that bacillary dysentery precipitates acute beriberi. Intestinal absorption of thiamin involves passive and active components (Rindu & Ventura 1972) and could be disrupted by disturbed intestinal function and changes in bowel flora.

We found abnormal thiamin status to be associated with both nutritional neglect and infection in 91 patients aged 61–91 on admission to hospital (Figure 7.2). The effects were additive for 57% of patients with nutritional neglect without infection, had an abnormal thiamin status (Thiamin pyrophosphate (TPP) effect > 20% [TK–AC > 1.2]) compared to 81% when infection was also present.

In patients who developed an infection during admission there was a significant increase in the TPP effect (Table 7.6). The change in TPP effect was greatest in those patients where infection was associated with an acute confusional state. None of the patients was given thiamin supplements but the biochemical abnormalities tended to return to normal when the infection was treated.

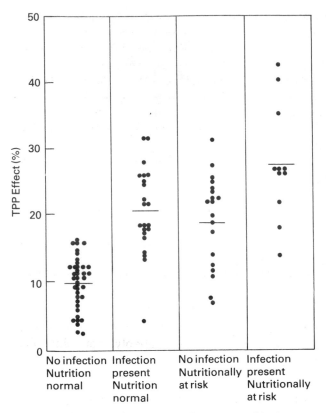

Fig. 7.2   Thiamin status (TPP effect %) in elderly patients on admission to hospital. TPP effect is greater in patients who have an infection or are nutritionally at risk.

Other water soluble vitamins

The effects of infestation with the fish tapeworm *Diphyllobothrium latumon* on vitamin B$_{12}$ status is well documented. Anaemic patients with hookworm infections tend to absorb folate poorly and had low serum vitamin B$_{12}$ levels (Layrisse *et al*. 1959). It is suggested that respiratory infections may precipitate megaloblastic anaemias in monkeys maintained on a low folate diet (Scrimshaw *et al*. 1968).

Table 7.6 Changes in TPP effect with infection and confusion.

Infection	Confusion	No	TPP Effect % (Mean and Range)			
			Basal*	Day 0	Day 4	Day 8
Absent	Absent	33	–	8 (5–15)	10 (5–16)	10 (5–15)
Present	Absent	9	7 (2–14)	18 (8–26)	16 (7–22)	11 (5–18)
Absent	Present	9	9 (4–14)	12 (4–18)	13 (4–21)	14 (10–17)
Present	Present	14	14 (3–23)	27 (18–32)	18 (2–40)	16 (2–28)

* Basal refers to value prior to onset of confusion
** Day 0 refers to day of onset of confusion or diagnosis of infections

Children with gastroenteritis have been found to have low levels of pyridoxine (Araya *et al.* 1975) as well as of other vitamins, but these changes are probably not clinically significant.

ATYPICAL PRESENTATION OF INFECTION IN THE ELDERLY IN RELATION TO NUTRITION

Confusion

A number of mechanisms predispose the elderly to confusion (Table 7.7) which is the presenting feature in approximately 40% of admissions to a geriatric unit. Changes in mental state are commonly seen with infection in the elderly. Infection is known to precipitate Wernicke's encephalopathy in alcoholics and could also cause confusion in the elderly by precipitating thiamin deficiency in those who already have a marginal thiamin status.

Table 7.7   Factors predisposing the
elderly to confusion.

Factors
Chronic organic brain syndrome
Sensory impairment
Environment
Isolation
Sleep disturbance
Drugs

We found that the change in TPP effect with infection was
greatest in those who initially had marginal thiamin status and it
was this group who were most likely to develop an acute confusional state (Table 7.6). There is also an association between the
development of abnormal thiamin status and postoperative confusion in elderly patients undergoing femoral neck surgery
(Older & Dickerson 1982).

Intracerebral thiamin levels are maintained by homeostatic
mechanisms as discussed in chapter 6. The elderly may be particularly vulnerable to disruption of these mechanisms (Threatt
et al. 1971) and may therefore be more vulnerable to the
neurological complications of thiamin deficiency. Our and Older
and Dickerson's observations on confusional episodes support
this proposition. It is possible that prophylactic administration of
thiamin supplements to 'at risk' elderly patients may modify the
frequency and course of toxic confusional states precipitated by
infection.

Pyrexia

The frequent absence of a pyrexial response to infection in old
age is well recognised. A defect in one or more of the several
stages in the production of fever (Figure 7.3) may be present.

Healthy well nourished elderly subjects appear to be able to
produce endogenous pyrogen normally (Junes et al. 1984).
Protein energy malnutrition may impair the pyrexial response by
reducing production of endogenous pyrogen (Hoffman-Goetz &

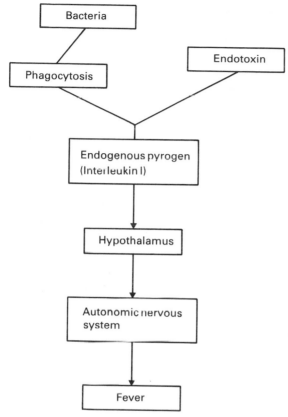

Fig. 7.3 Stages in the development of pyrexia.

Kluger 1979; Hoffman-Goetz *et al.* 1981) but refeeding by hyper-alimentation reverses these abnormalities. The profound effect of avitaminosis on neutrophil and lymphocyte function described earlier may also interfere with endogenous pyrogen production.

CONCLUSION

Vitamin deficiency has profound effects on host defence mechanisms. It is reasonable to suggest therefore that the vitamin deficiencies which are common in the elderly may both predispose them to infection and modify the clinical picture.

Changes in measures of vitamin status with infection have been documented. There is some circumstantial evidence to link changes in thiamin status with infection and confusion in the elderly but the clinical significance of this finding remains to be established.

8   Assessment of Cognitive Function in the Elderly

R.J. Ancill and A.C. Carr

The measurement of the function of the brain is presently, and for the foreseeable future likely to remain, an inexact science. Our models of brain function are either related to grossly indirect parameters such as electrical activity, or to complex pieces of behaviour. Although we have tried to limit the problem by restricting ourselves to measuring cognitive function we have not succeeded in defining or establishing parameters which determine any particular function or are sensitive enough to change. Whitehead (1982) highlighted these problems by asking what it is that it would be appropriate to measure, particularly in those patients who are known to have cognitive dysfunction such as is found in dementia. It was felt that the process to be measured should be of practical relevance, a direct measurement of a known function or ability, and should measure a function known to be impaired at a given level of illness.

The organic brain illness that most commonly requires our attention is dementia and it is desirable that assessments of cognitive function not only assesses the severity of the condition, but also helps to discriminate among the differential diagnoses. Lishman (1978) described dementia as a syndrome characterised by 'acquired global impairment of memory or personality but without impairment of consciousness'.

Unfortunately, in this severe and progressive organic brain disease virtually all functions can be affected, which may lead to the patient being substantially non-assessable by conventional means. On the other hand, at the mildest, and probably the more treatable end of the disease spectrum, standard tests are likely to give normal or ambiguous results. They are certainly not particularly sensitive to the amounts of change that might be expected with the range of interventions that we have now, or can expect to have in the next few years.

Psychologists have tended to concentrate their efforts on the assessment of memory function in this type of patient as it is generally believed that memory impairment is one of the earliest and commonest signs. However, Heaton *et al.* (1978) pointed out that although many studies have shown that the patient's performance on memory tests may differentiate those with organic brain syndromes from those with other psychiatric disorders, the majority contain serious methodological flaws, therefore their clinical usefulness is suspect. Although more recently Coughlan and Hollows (1984) have suggested that memory tests can have a useful role in discriminating between organic disorders and depression, it is still generally true that standard tests appear to be of limited use. Furthermore, there is substantial disagreement amongst psychologists as to the nature of the memory deficit and as to what particular type of test should be used. Davies and Mumford (1984) have recently suggested that the memory deficit found in dementia can be better explained as a failure of processing when new information is acquired, rather than a failure to retrieve. It is therefore not surprising that there are a plethora of 'tests'.

Blessed (1980) observed that when using the standard combination of tests with 244 elderly hospitalised patients, those with dementia scored significantly worse than those with acute brain syndromes, who in turn scored worse than those with medical (non brain) illness. However, Blessed draws attention to the fact that one particular patient with proven dementia scored virtually within the normal range and that depressed patients scored particularly poorly. It must be remembered that few elderly patients will present with 'pure' illness, but will rather have multisystem problems which makes interpretation of test scores even more difficult.

Tests of cognitive dysfunction fall into 3 main groups which are (1) Performance (2) Conversational and (3) Psychometric. None of these categories has a particularly tight definition and they all suffer from the problem that they attempt to assess extremely complex tasks involving many functions and abilities involving perception, attention, processing, recall and expression. However it is worth considering these groups, looking at what is currently done together with their advantages and disadvantages.

TESTS OF COGNITIVE DYSFUNCTION

Performance & behavioural

Observation

Several scales have been devised (e.g. CAPE, GRUMPIE, PADL) but perhaps the most commonly used one is the Clifton Assessment Procedure in the Elderly (CAPE) behaviour rating scale which consists of 3 elements, namely the information-orientation, mental ability and psychomotor tasks. The person administering the CAPE requires little training and the patient is likely to understand tasks which tend to assess natural and motivated behaviour such as dressing, and it is quite possible to do multiple trials in order to allow assessment of optimal performance. However, there will be a marked influence from physical and perceptual deficits. The patient will either succeed or fail on a given task, thus rendering the score somewhat insensitive to subtle changes. The motivation of the patient may be affected by the 'sick role', dependence and other factors such as depression. Multiple abilities and functions are involved, and the CAPE is therefore used primarily for a global assessment and is not particularly sensitive to change over time.

Tests

These tests are aimed at defining specific dysfunctions such as the dyspraxias through various tasks such as drawing and matchstick construction. They require trained staff, but patients generally comprehend the task and multiple trials are possible. Again performance is likely to be affected by physical and perceptual problems and comprehension depends on hearing. The results are usually measured as success or failure and patients sometimes find failing on these tests humiliating, which leads to decreased motivation and subsequent poorer performance. These tests can be useful for qualitative detection of suspected brain lesions but they are not capable of measuring change.

Conversational tests

This approach involves the patient in conversation although the interview tends to be a structured one. Comprehension of proverbs, Babcock sentences, time-place orientation and general knowledge are among the more common tests that are used and form part of assessment procedures such as the CAPE and the Gresham. These assessments can be done by non-skilled personnel and the tests themselves are easily comprehensible. Provided that the patient is not dysphasic, the results are independent of physical handicaps. Furthermore, no special test materials are required. However, these tests are not easily repeatable and they are influenced by the patient's mental state. The tests depend on hearing and speech and in patients with minimal disease, questions can appear to be humiliating. Being structured in nature, tho questions may be inappropriate for patients whose recent status has made them ill-informed about current events or dates. The only measure is accuracy and it is restricted to memory recall which is known to be affected by the educational level of the patient. These tests may be particularly inappropriate in immigrants. Nevertheless, this type of assessment is probably the most widely used and the results correlate well with other tests.

Psychometric tests

Tests in this category are designed to measure specific abilities and functions and they require skilled personnel to deliver the tests as well as specific materials. These tests assess such aspects of cognitive function as learning (with wordlists, paired-association), memory (famous faces, famous events), logical thinking (sorting tests), reaction time, and a whole variety of further tests that are designed to examine all the neurological and psychological parameters that have so far been defined. These tests allow detailed and accurate measurements of speed, learning, retention and error. Repeated testing can often be used to monitor for progress and fluctuations and there is a significant degree of inter-test correlation. Various different functions can be examined and compared and the results tend to be relatively unaffected by education, culture and recent status. Many of these tests, however, are still substantially qualitative, determining loss or preservation of function and often what is being measured may have little clinical relevance or neurological foundation. Psychometric tests are often difficult to explain to impaired patients and rely on perceptual preservation and dexterity. The results are susceptible to distraction and chance emotive associations. They can also be greatly affected by concentration, attention and other motivational factors. The simple automation of such traditional tests has failed to improve the situation significantly.

This chapter is an attempt to provide an overview of what is currently available and as such it can be seen that the situation is hardly satisfactory. Most assessments tend to answer a qualitative question such as whether or not the patient is demented and are of little value in determining the severity of the condition, or of indicating changes that might be brought about by chemotherapy or improved nutrition. It may be that there are several clinical manoeuvres that might be of some benefit to these patients, but the tests are too insensitive to detect small amounts of change and may therefore lead the clinician to decide that a given treatment has no effect and abandon that treatment when a real effect might have been achieved (false negative errors).

The ideal assessment should be repeatable and give quantitative results. One approach could be to look at gradients of learning that would allow examination of parameters that were independent of the actual test.

Carr *et al.* (1982) demonstrated that microcomputers could be used to deliver assessments to psychogeriatric patients. This and further work has shown that many 'untreatable' elderly patients can be assessed with a computer when certain criteria are met.

1 The brightness of the screen must be raised to counteract retinal cell loss in the aged eye.
2 Audio cues are necessary to maximise attention.
3 The speed of visual information must be reduced by around a factor of 3.
4 A specialised response instrument should be used, e.g. touch-sensitive screens, large key-keyboards.

5   Positive feedback is important even when errors are made avoiding 'catastrophic' reactions.

6   Even when progressively more difficult tests are being used, there should be regular easy items.

This approach opens up the potential of using automated techniques that would not require the presence of highly trained and expensive personnel, as well as allowing a greater range of assessments to be made. It is particularly important to ensure that the patient is capable of perceiving accurately material featured in the tests: failure to do this may lead to the confusing of a perceptual dysfunction with a cognitive one. Preliminary work using the Maudsley Automated Tests for the Elderly (MATE) has suggested that such a technique has potential although the problem still remains as to what assessments should be delivered. One way around this problem may be to use a micro-computer and any test that involves multiple abilities, modify the test to add one additional function, administer the test with and without the added function and then compare the results of the learning curves of both tests. The difference between tests should be a reasonable measure of this additional function. An example of this would be a simple maze-learning task compared with the same maze rotated 90 degrees. Such modifications are simple to execute on a computer, which has the advantage of saving and analysing the results as well.

The development of such sophisticated approaches make it reasonable to expect that future assessment of cognitive function in elderly patients will reflect the effects of treatment and environmental manipulations.

9 Nutrition and Dementia

D.E. Thomas, K.O. Chung-a-on, M.H. Briscoe,
S.F. Tidmarsh, J.W.T. Dickerson and
D.M. Shaw

INTRODUCTION

Dementia is a syndrome of global disturbance of higher mental functions in an alert patient (Marsden 1978). Its prevalence has been estimated to be 2.4% among 65–69 years-olds compared with 22% for those aged 80 and over (Kay *et al.* 1964; Kay *et al.* 1970). Admissions to hospital for dementia exceed those for all other disabilities in old age (Kay *et al.* 1970). This condition alone makes heavy and rising demands on social and hospital services as well as causing tremendous personal and family distress.

The term 'senile dementia' is taken to include Alzheimer's disease and senile dementia of Alzheimer type. Although there are differences between these two conditions, their similarities are many and pending further evidence, it is usual to consider them together.

This chapter examines the possibility that there may be an association between senile dementia and nutrition. Nutritional deficiences are not uncommon in old people particularly those in institutions, but not all old people in the community and not even all those in institutions, become demented. It is therefore necessary to examine the hypothesis that nutritional deficiences may cause dementia or exacerbate its underlying pathology.

INSTITUTIONALISATION AND AGEING

Discussion of the possible effects of nutrition on brain function in the elderly, and on the dementing process, is likely to be confounded by the fact that dementing old people have often been in hospital for sometime and have become 'institutionalised'. Any deficiencies in the provision of food and in its nutrient content will have left their mark on the patients. Vir and Love (1979) reported that the nutrient intake of old people in institutions was lower than that of those in the community and although clinical deficiency was rare among in-patients, sub-clinical deficiences were common. However, others (MacLennan *et al.* 1975; Asplund *et al.* 1981) have reported adequate intakes of energy and protein by longstay patients. It seems likely that the effects of institutionalisation will vary and that the health of the patient (or resident) may be a factor influencing nutritional intake.

Crosssectional studies purporting to show a decrease in nutrient intake with increasing age must be interpreted with caution. It is necessary to demonstrate a change in the nutrient of individuals as they age, i.e. a longitudinal change. The results of such a study by Stanton and Exton-Smith (1970) showed that a decrease in food intake occurred only in individuals whose health score had decreased. These findings were in agreement with previous studies from the United States. Stanton and Exton-Smith's study involved individuals with somatic disease and it seems that the effect of food intake is unlikely to be a simple one but rather the result of a downwardly directed spiral with reduced nutrient intake exacerbating ill health.

The spiral effect may be equally evident in individuals with mental disease. Elderly women with dementia have been reported (Morgan & Hullin 1982) to have lower body weights than women with affective disorders and schizophrenia. This difference in weight was not related to length of stay in hospital and there was no evidence that it was due to malnutrition. They concluded that low body weight was possibly a marker for those persons likely to need hospital care.

We will return to the possible involvement of energy and protein nutriture in dementia after discussing the possible role played by vitamins.

VITAMINS OF THE B-GROUP

Many vitamins of the B-group, particularly thiamin, nicotinic acid, pyridoxine, folic acid (Reynolds *et al.* 1971; Wells 1965) and vitamin B_{12} play important roles in brain metabolism and their deficiencies are associated with neurological or psychiatric diseases so that it is tempting to consider that deficiencies of these vitamins may be involved in the aetiology of dementia in old people. However, the evidence appears somewhat contradictory for whilst Kershaw (1967) found no biochemical evidence of thiamin or nicotinic acid deficiency in patients with senile dementia, Carney *et al.* (1979) reported that thiamin and pyridoxine deficiencies were common in 154 newly admitted psychiatric patients of which a proportion had senile dementia. There is accumulating evidence that low thiamin status is common among the elderly (see Chapter 5). Katakity *et al.* (1983) found evidence of low thiamin status in 9 out of 12 patients in a geriatric hospital and in 3 patients with pneumonia, who became acutely confused, the TPP effect (Brin 1964) declined progressively with treatment as the confusional state resolved. The conclusion that there was an association between mental confusion and thiamin deficiency accorded with an earlier report on post-operative confusion in elderly fracture patients (Older and Dickerson 1982; see also Chapter 7).

A number of investigators have considered the role of folic acid in relation to dementia. Strachan and Henderson (1967) described an improvement in the mental state of two patients with senile dementia following treatment with folate. The cause of folate deficiency in these patients appeared to be insufficient intake of the vitamin.

Batata *et al.* (1967) studied a group of patients newly admitted to a geriatric department, and found a high prevalence of low serum folic acid concentrations without an associated megaloblastic anaemia especially in those with organic brain disease. An enquiry into their diet led to the conclusion that the majority had poor intakes of folate, although recall of their diet might have been unreliable. Serum levels of folate do not correlate with red cell folate (MacLennan *et al.* 1975) and probably provide information on the recent intake of folate (see Chapter 4) which in the individuals studied by Batata *et al.* (1967) might have been lower due to illness before admission to hospital. The red cell folate level may be a more valid measurement in that it may reflect long term folate status more accurately.

The explanation offered by Sneath *et al.* (1973) for their association of low folate and dementia was that dementia leads to a poor dietary intake and in turn folate deficiency, rather than the converse. In the authors view, it is premature to make this claim, and the possibility that folate deficiency itself may lead to impaired mental function should continue to be explored.

Perhaps it should not be assumed that bone marrow is more sensitive to lack of folate than is the central nervous system. However, in severe cases both may be affected. Anand (1964) described a patient with megaloblastic anaemia, myelopathy, impairment of memory and moderate dementia of frontal lobe type, who showed no response to vitamin B_{12}, but who improved in all aspects after taking folate. Further discussion of the association of folate and vitamin B_{12} with mental function will be found in Chapters 3 and 5.

We have not been able to find any reports of investigation of riboflavin and pyridoxine status specifically in patients with senile dementia.

Vitamin C

Clinically induced lack of vitamin C has produced personality changes, including 'hysteria' and depression (Hughes 1982). One possible link between mood and lack of vitamin C is the reduction in activity of dopamine β-hydroxylase in scurvy. This enzyme is ascorbic acid-dependent and it converts 3,4di-hydroxy-phenethylamine (dopamine) to noradrenaline, a neurotransmitter likely to be implicated in depressed states. These links between vitamin C and some neurotransmitters make ascorbic acid of interest when investigating the patient with senile dementia, since biogenic amine pathways are not normal in dementia, dopamine levels are reduced (Rosser et al. 1984) and depressive symptoms are common in this condition.

Exton-Smith (1978) claimed that in the elderly, sub-clinical deficiencies of folate and vitamins C and D were the most common (see Chapter 5). This has been supported by Kataria et al. (1965) and Taylor (1968), who found poor vitamin C status in elderly patients in a geriatric ward, compared with those living at home. It is very difficult to ascribe a specific role for vitamin C deficiency in senile dementia. There is little evidence that it is more common in patients with this condition than in other elderly patients in psychiatric institutions.

However, in a recent study of plasma vitamin C concentrations in patients in a psychiatric ward Schorah et al. (1983) found low values in patients with senile dementia which they were unable to explain. Intakes were not assessed but other patients consuming the same diet had higher plasma concentrations.

The major cause of low vitamin C status is likely to be a low intake. This can be due to poor food choice but it is also exacerbated by the vulnerability of the vitamin to losses during the storage, preparation and cooking of vegetables. Thus, Eddy (1963) suggested that 13% of the calculated value of vitamin C as estimated from food tables was lost in the cooking of garden peas. Platt *et al.* (1963) described losses of 45–60% of vitamin C in hospital vegetables when they were soaked in water overnight. Black *et al.* (1983) found that the mean analytical values for cooked vegetables were generally close to current food table values (Paul & Southgate 1979), although the range was wide. This emphasised the fact that food table values are averages and do not necessarily represent the composition of actual items consumed. The authors own studies at Whitchurch Hospital (Table 9.1) showed that potato lost 92% of its vitamin C during preparation, cooking and service (Thomas *et al.* 1985).

Table 9.1 Percentage loss of ascorbic acid by potato at Whitchurch Hospital between preparation and serving.

Time	State of potato	Ascorbic acid mg/100 g potato	% loss
09.00 hours	raw	10.00	–
11.15 hours	immediately after cooking	5.11	49
12.30 hours	when served	0.89	92

Neurotransmitters, amino acids and dementia

There is clear evidence of deficiency of cholinergic transmission in the brains of patients with dementia of the Alzheimer type (see Bowen & Davison 1984). Increasing the amount of choline or lecithin in the diet increases the concentration of acetylcholine in the plasma and in the brain (Cohen & Wurtman 1976; Lancet 1980). Experiments in rats have shown that the converse is also true, i.e. decreasing dietary choline decreases brain acetycholine. It is clearly tempting to consider the possibility that increasing the choline intake would lead to an improvement in the mental health of patients with Alzheimer's disease. However, the results of giving high choline or lecithin diets to patients have been disappointing (Bartus et al. 1982) possibly because of sensitive homeostatic mechanisms in the brain which tend to reduce the acutely-raised concentrations of acetycholine (Ferris et al. 1979).

Interest has been recently focussed on the possibility that deterioration of serotoninergic neurones may be involved in senile dementia. This possibility is attractive because of the evidence that serotonin synthesis can be affected by supply of the precursor, tryptophan and the manipulation of other factors which modify the transport of tryptophan into the brain.

Some patients with senile dementia may have an intestinal defect which reduces their ability to absorb tryptophan (Lehmann 1070, Lehmann et al. 1981). When large amounts of tryptophan (100 mg/kg body weight) were given with l-dopa, a competitor for absorption across the gut mucosa, it was possible to distinguish two populations one with a 'normal' rise in plasma tryptophan concentrations and another with a 'reduced' rise.

Giving a high protein diet with supplements of tryptophan resulted in clinical improvement in those individuals who had been diagnosed as having senile dementia and who had 'low' plasma tryptophan levels following the 'loading' test. In addition, Lehmann showed that amounts of urinary indican were enhanced in these patients, showing that tryptophan had not been absorbed adequately from the gut, and the amino acid had passed on to the large intestine where it had been converted to indican, which was excreted in the urine.

The results suggested the presence of a subgroup of patients with senile dementia with decreased ability to absorb amino acids from the gut, whose condition might be improved by dietary supplements.

Using a lower test dose of tryptophan and no 'competitor', Shaw et al. (1981) were unable to demonstrate a bimodal population with 'normal' and 'low' plasma levels, although the range of plasma levels achieved was much wider in the patients than in a control group.

There was, however, a highly significant decrease in the fasting levels of plasma tryptophan and in the 'tryptophan ratio' (the ratio of the concentration of tryptophan to the sum of the concentrations of tyrosine, phenylalanine, leucine, isoleucine and valine). There was also a significant decrease in the ratio of concentration of tyrosine to that of the sum of tryptophan, phenylalanine, leucine, isoleucine and valine in plasma. Thus the supply of both these amino acids to the brain overnight (while fasting) might have been at risk in patients suffering from senile dementia. It follows that protein synthesis in the brains of these individuals might be reduced by imbalance in the supply of amino acids.

It seems possible that an impaired supply of tryptophan to the brain may be incriminated in senile dementia and several factors can affect this supply. The level of non-protein bound tryptophan is important in the transport process and can be modified by drugs and non-esterified fatty acids (NEFA) (Curzon *et al.* 1973). The insulin response to dietary carbohydrate is also important. These various factors have been examined (Thomas *et al.* unpublished) in a group of 29 patients with senile dementia matched with appropriate controls. The concentrations of total tryptophan in the plasma of the patients with senile dementia were significantly lower than in the controls and this was accounted for by lower concentrations of the protein-bound fraction. Lower concentrations of albumin and NEFA were also found in the patients but there was a significant correlation between the concentrations of NEFA and free tryptophan in the controls. Such a correlation was not found in the patients. It seems possible that the lower concentrations of tryptophan in the patients could have been due to an absorptive defect for the amino acid as suggested by Lehmann's work.

Tryptophan is converted to nicotinamide via the kynurenine pathway but there was no evidence of increased metabolism of tryptophan down this pathway in our patients. Plasma concentrations of insulin were similar in patients and controls and thus there was no evidence that there was likely to have been any change in the cellular/extracellular distribution of the neutral amino acids that compete for transport into the brain.

If the low values of tryptophan in patients with senile dementia are to be explained by defective absorption of tryptophan from the gut it seems unlikely that the defect will affect only the absorption of this amino acid. Furthermore it seemed possible that nutritional deficiencies might exacerbate the dementia even if not involved in the aetiology of the structural defects that occur in the brain in this condition. Previous work reviewed earlier in this chapter was not directed specifically to this problem.

DIETARY INTAKE AND NUTRITIONAL STATUS IN DEMENTIA

Energy intake

Undernutrition is thought to be common and obesity rare in patients in psychogeriatric wards. In the study in Cardiff (Thomas *et al.* 1985) the authors of this chapter found (Table 9.2) lower energy intakes in the 23 patients than in the 23 age/sex matched healthy controls living at home. This finding must be seen against the background of activity seen in some patients in dementia. A proportion are restless, and the ambulant ones spend much of their day walking around. It is likely therefore that their energy expenditure is greater than that of their healthy counterparts.

Although 87% of the patients had energy intakes below the RDA (DHSS 1979b), they ate all the food presented to them. Some attempted to steal food from other patients and appeared to have no preferences for any foods. On the relatively rare occasions when food was not eaten, the patient could either not masticate it or was 'in a mood'. As discussed above, the body weight of patients with dementia tends to be low when compared for instance with that of elderly patients with affective disorders of schizophrenia (Morgan & Hullin 1982). Although the RDA for the healthy elderly is sometimes considered to be too high, this may not be true of patients with senile dementia.

Vitamin C

Although the mean calculated intake of vitamin C by the patients exceeded the recommended dietary intake (RDA) (DHSS 1979b) evidence already discussed suggests that these valus are spuriously high. This conclusion was supported by the finding

(Table 9.3) of a lower mean plasma concentration of vitamin C with a greater number of patients compared with controls having values below the accepted 'safe' lower limit. The authors of this chapters' findings suggest that there may be a valid case for supplementation with this vitamin. The fact that there is no evidence of scurvy in patients with senile dementia is not a reason for omitting supplements. Muscle weakness, for instance, is caused by sub-clinical ascorbic acid deficiency (Hughes 1982).

Thiamin and riboflavin

The requirements for thiamin and riboflavin are related to the energy intake. About a fifth of all these authors' (Thomas *et al.*) subjects (patients and controls) were receiving less than the RDA of thiamin, and 36% of the controls and 38% of the patients had biochemical evidence of thiamin deficiency on the basis of elevated values for transketolase activation. This finding agrees with the values in other studies of geriatric patients (Older & Dickerson 1982; Katakity *et al.* 1983) and is clearly not restricted to patients with senile dementia. A number of factors may contribute to the appearance of thiamin deficiency such as destruction of thiamin during cooking, losses in the stomach due to the use of antacids (Dickerson 1978), and malabsorption.

Nicotinic Acid

Intake of nicotinic acid was adequate and only one of the control subjects had biochemical evidence of deficiency. The mean N^1 methylnicotinamide/creatinine ratio in urine was similar in patients and controls.

Pyridoxine

Pyridoxine is present in a wide variety of foods with no food being a particularly rich source. Assuming an allowance of 1 mg/day, significantly more patients (64%) than controls (43%) had a low intake, but only 5% of the patients and none of the controls had biochemical evidence of a deficiency of this vitamin.

Table 9.2 Daily nutrient intake of 23 patients with senile dementia and 23 control subjects (9 males and 14 females in each group).

	Group	Mean	SD	'p' value†	RDA*	% below RDA	Chi² (p) value
Energy (kcal)	Senile dements	1540	± 240 ⎫	<0.01	M 2275	87 ⎫	<0.001
	Controls	1890	± 520 ⎭		F 1750	39 ⎭	
Protein (g)	Senile dements	59	± 9	<0.02	M 57	13 ⎫	NS
	Controls	67	± 13		F 44.5	4 ⎭	
Tryptophan (mg)	Senile dements	780	± 153	NS			
	Controls	836	± 186				
Ascorbic acid (mg)	Senile dements	35	± 10	<0.02	30	39	
	Controls	47	± 20			17	
Thiamin (mg)	Senile dements	1.0	± 0.3	NS	M 0.9	30	
	Controls	1.1	± 0.3		F 0.7	8	
Riboflavin (mg)	Senile dements	1.8	± 0.5	NS	M 1.6	27	
	Controls	1.7	± 0.6		F 1.3	39	

Table 9.2 — *cont'd*

	Group	Mean	SD	'p' value†	RDA*	% below RDA	Chi² (p) value
Nicotinic acid (mg equiv.)	Senile dements	24 ±	5.9 ⎫	<0.003	M 18	0	
	Controls	31 ±	8.6 ⎬		F 15	0	
Pyridoxine (mg)	Senile dements	1.0 ±	0.2 ⎫	NS	1mg**	64	
	Controls	1.1 ±	0.3 ⎬			43	
Folic acid (µg)	Senile dements	141 ±	34 ⎫	NS	200***	100	
	Controls	140 ±	40 ⎬			91	

  * Recommended daily allowance (DHSS 1979)
 ** USA Recommended daily allowance
*** Recommended daily allowance (DHSS 1969)
  † NS not significant.

Table 9.3 Vitamin status of 23 patients with senile dementia and of 23 control subjects.

Variable	Group	limit of normal	Mean		SD	'p' value†	% below normal value	Chi² 'p' value
Ascorbic acid plasma (mg/100 ml)	Senile dements	> 0.4	0.46	±	0.29	0.003	46	<0.01
	Controls		0.77	±	0.36		9	
Ascorbic acid buffy coat (µg/10^8 cells)	Senile dements	> 18	35	±	14	NS	10	NS
	Controls		42	±	18		9	
Thiamin *TPP effect	Senile dements	< 15	21	±	3	NS	38	NS
	Controls		34	±	70		36	
Riboflavin *FAD effect	Senile dements	< 76	32	±	20	NS	0	NS
	Controls		30	±	14		0	
Pyridoxine *PLP effect	Senile dements	<130	54	±	8	NS	5	NS
	Controls		59	±	4		0	
Folic acid serum µg/ml	Senile dements	> 2	5.1	±	0	NS	5	NS
	Controls		6.7	±	3		0	

Table 9.3 — *cont'd*

Variable	Group	limit of normal	Mean	SD	'p' value†	% below normal value	Chi² 'p' value
Erythrocyte µg/ml	Senile dements	<100	198	± 101	0.05	0	NS
	Controls		308	± 201		6	

* TPP Effect, FAD effect and PLP effect
Results shown are (stimulated — basal) enzyme activity as % of basal activity

	Enzyme	Stimulated by
TPP effect	Transketolase	Thiamin pyrophosphate
FAD effect	Glutathione reductase	Flavin adenine dinucleotide
PLP effect	Aspartate amino transferase	Pyridoxal 5 phosphate

† NS not significant.

Folic acid

There are a number of sources of error in currently used assay techniques for measuring folate in foods (Bates *et al.* 1982). The availability of the various forms and conjugates that are measured is not fully understood. Paul & Southgate (1979) state in their introduction to the McCance and Widdowson Food Tables that the estimates of folic acid in foods in the 4th edition will need revision in the future, and that this should be borne in mind when assessing dietary intakes. Official recommendations for folate intakes (DHSS 1979b) tend to be very much higher than current intakes, and are not included in later reprints of the recommendations (see Table 2.1). We have adopted the previously recommended figure of 200 μg as a yardstick for assessing folate intakes.

Almost all the subjects were receiving less than 200 μg of folic acid per day and serum folate levels were normal. Since cases of dementia due to folic acid deficiency have been described (Sneath *et al.* 1973), the findings in the present study of lower red cell folate levels in dementia patients was of interest, particularly since folate synthesis, transport and metabolism might be implicated in the pathogenesis of a variety of neurological and psychiatric disorders (Levi & Waxman 1975; Reynolds 1976). Folate deficiency may effect serotonin synthesis via its effect on the synthesis of a methyl donor S-adensoyl-L-methionine which has been shown to increase the turnover of serotonin in rat brain (Algeri *et al.* 1979).

CONCLUSIONS

The fact that dementia occurs in old people and that the demented become longstay patients in psychiatric hospital complicates the nutritional picture. There is presently no clear evidence that any nutritional deficiency is found specifically in such patients though there are suggestions that folic acid deficiency may play a role in some patients. Deficiencies of intake cannot necessarily be interpreted as evidence of nutritional deficiency and they may be a consequence, rather than a cause of dementia. The possible inter-relationships between nutrition and brain structure and metabolism in dementia are doubtlessly complex and it may be that the diseased brain is more sensitive to changes in the availability of nutrients. In order to establish a role of nutrient deficiency as a cause of dementia it would be necessary to carry out longitudinal assessments in individuals during worsening of brain function. Investigation is further complicated by the fact that clinical assessments and differentiation are imprecise. It would seem necessary to identify a group of patients with early senile dementia and to assess their response to tryptophan and vitamin supplements.

10 Nutrition of Elderly Patients with Cancer

by *Professor J.W.T. Dickerson*

INTRODUCTION

Many patients with cancer lose weight during the course of their illness and this is often the first indication of malignancy. The syndrome of anorexia, weakness, wasting and weight loss known as 'cachexia' appears to be independent of tumour bulk (Calman 1982) and has been attributed to the cancer specific changes in metabolism (Lawson *et al.* 1982) due to the production of tissue-toxic substances (Theologides 1979) and interference with nutrition of the host tissues (White 1945). In spite of indications that changes in metabolism in the cancer patient are cancer specific, it seems that the consequent changes in indices of nutritional status are not different from those in undernourished patients with non-malignant disease (Lennard *et al.* 1983).

Anorexia in the cancer patient is often exacerbated by treatment such as chemotherapy and radiotherapy and the added complications of nausea and vomiting together with mucositis, ageusia and xerostomia all militate against the patient being able to consume an adequate amount of food (Fig 10.1; Ivey 1982). The consequent malnutrition may interfere with anti-tumour therapy and impair the patient's chances of recovery.

METABOLIC CHANGES

Changes in protein and fat metabolism reported in patients with cancer have been reviewed elsewhere (Dickerson 1984a). There is evidence that oncological disease is associated with an increased rate of protein turnover, an increased rate of protein synthesis in the liver, a decreased rate of protein synthesis in skeletal muscle and a simultaneous increase in net degradation of muscle protein. These changes are very similar to those reported in children with protein energy malnutrition (Alleyne *et*

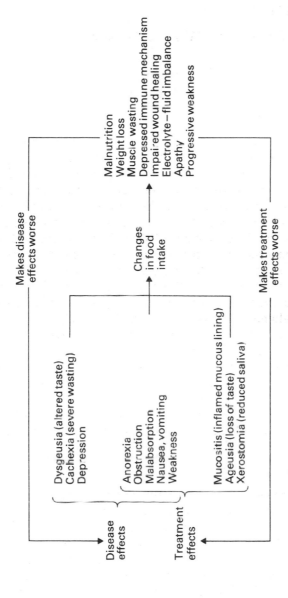

Fig. 10.1 Nutritional implications of cancer and cancer therapy.

al. 1977). Low albumin values are common in patients with cancer, but these cannot be assumed to indicate poor nutritional status until other causes have been excluded (Moore *et al.* 1982). Although cancer patients frequently lose body fat, it is not clear whether their fat metabolism is different from that in patients with other diseases in which nutrition is compromised. The basic defect may be a failure of homeostatic mechanisms possibly due to insulin insensitivity (Lundholm *et al.* 1978).

FEEDING THE PATIENT

From a practical point of view the feeding of cancer patients presents a challenge. Appetite is often poor, taste sensation may be deranged (DeWys & Walters 1975; Hall *et al.* 1980) and the patient is easily satisfied with small amounts of food. All these factors reduce the likelihood of the patient being able to consume sufficient food to restore, or even maintain body weight, and considerable skill and resourcefulness is necessary if they are to be overcome. Perhaps the most important factor in relation to oral feeding is the patient's own psychological reaction to his disease and its treatment. In a preliminary study of patients treated with radiotherapy appetite and psychological state were found to be correlated with each other and also with the amount of nurse-patient contact (Evans & Dickerson unpublished).

The nutritional problems of the cancer patient have attracted a great deal of attention (Dickerson 1983; 1984a) and there is discussion as to whether the nutritional management of these patients should differ from that of other malnourished patients (Buzby *et al.* 1980). Lennard *et al.* (1983) have concluded that nutritional support of cancer patients should follow the principles established (MacBurney & Wilmore 1981) for management of any malnourished patient since anthropometric and biochemical indices of nutritional status are similar in the two groups.

Advances in techniques of anaesthesia, surgery and intensive care have encouraged surgeons to undertake more extensive and crippling operations which may further threaten the patient's ability to maintain his nutritional status.

Long-term dependence on tube-feeding may be necessary in for instance, patients having surgery for head and neck cancer.

Enteral feeding through a jejunostomy is useful following oesophagectomy and reconstruction (Schattenkerk *et al.* 1984) and patients may be sent home with a jejunostomy pending reconstruction.

After major surgery nutritional advice and support for the patient and relatives must continue after the patient leaves hospital and the dietitian has a key role to play. The nutritional care team might be extended to include general practitioners and health visitors as well as relatives (Fig 10.2; Trodger 1082) and communication between hospital and community services is essential.

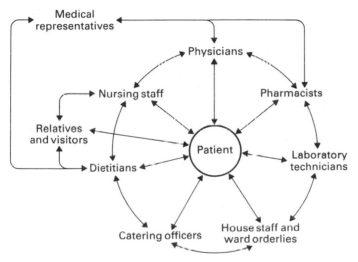

Fig. 10.2 Schematic outline of relationships between members of the nutrition team. (Reproduced with permission from Tredger (1982) *Nursing* **4**, 92–3.

Early reports particularly from the United States suggest that nutritional support might increase the effectiveness of anti-tumour therapy though these need to be confirmed by rigorous controlled studies. Malnourished patients are poor candidates for surgery, radiotherapy or chemotherapy but it is doubtful if improvements in nutritional status would improve their response to treatment (Brennan 1981). The possibility that nutritional support could improve the quality of life for patients with cancer merits further investigation, though it is difficult to devise methods of assessing subjective experience (Selby *et al.* 1984).

There is at present no satisfactory evidence that nutritional manipulation is an effective treatment for cancer and patients who are subjected to extreme dietary restrictions may become so severely malnourished as to preclude the use of conventional therapies. However it is understandable that patients who feel that orthodox therapy offers little hope may prefer to try dietary manipulation rather than endure the side-effects of chemo-therapy. Considerations of this sort may well account for the attraction of 'alternative' therapies and the patients may experi-ence a psychological uplift from the feeling that they are par-ticipating in their own treatment.

VITAMINS AND THE CANCER PATIENT

Most studies on the nutrition of the cancer patient and indeed on other critically ill patients have concentrated on the provision of energy and protein and less attention has been paid to their trace element and vitamin requirements. Deficiencies of a number of vitamins are common in patients with cancer (Table 10.1; Soukop & Calman 1979). It may well be that vitamin metabolism is deranged in patients with some kinds of cancer. Patients with breast cancer and particularly those with skeletal metastases appear to have a considerably increased requirement for vitamin C (Basu *et al.* 1974). Subsequent studies have shown dif-ferences in the response to a 3 g loading doses of ascorbic acid in patients with breast cancer and those with non-cancerous breast disease. Although both showed a normal rise in plasma ascorbic acid levels the cancer patients showed a smaller rise in leucocyte ascorbic acid levels (Poulter *et al.* 1985).

Cameron and Pauling (1978) suggested that high doses of ascorbic acid could prolong the life of patients with advanced cancer though others have not been able to repeat their results. However since Pauling suggested that ascorbic acid might exert its beneficial effect by stimulating the bodies own defence mechanisms it might be argued that the value of megadose ascorbic acid in cancer has not been fairly tested until it has

Table 10.1 Nutritional abnormalities in cancer patients (from Soukop & Calman).

	120 Cancer patients (%)	70 Hospital patients (%)
Anaemia	49	14
Low plasma retinol	15	3
Low plasma carotene	15	3
Thiamin deficient	37	16
Low leucocyte ascorbic acid	71	31
Abnormal folate	23	7
Abnormal B_{12}	0	0
Serum albumin > 30 g/l	20	3
Weight loss > 15%	45	1

been tried in patients who have refused radiotherapy and chemotherapy and whose immune system is intact (Dickerson 1981). Preliminary observations on patients with Paget's disease of bone suggest that ascorbic acid might be of use for the relief of bone pain in patients with skeletal metastases (Basu *et al.* 1978). Deficiencies of many vitamins can impair brain function (see Chapter 6) and vitamin supplementation might improve quality of life by correcting these disturbances.

A disturbing possibility that ascorbic acid supplements might stimulate tumour growth is raised by the observation that lung tumours contain higher concentrations of vitamin C than normal tissue and may have a high requirement for this vitamin (Anthony & Schorah 1982).

Cytotoxic drugs may increase the requirements for some vitamins. Studies in rats suggest that Vinblastine increases the metabolism of retinol. The drug 5-fluorouracil when given alone or in combination with other cytotoxics decreases the thiamin status in four weeks (Aksoy *et al.* 1980). Further work is necessary to establish whether patients taking this drug would derive any benefit from thiamin supplementation. Cancer chemotherapy often involves courses of drugs separated by treatment-free days and with one such regime (intermittent Vinblastine and Bleomycin for metastatic testicular teratoma) we found fluctuations in vitamin status with the treatment cycle (Atukorala et al. 1982).

Vitamin A and the prevention of malignancy

Retinol and carotene have attracted particular attention in relation to cancer (Peto et al. 1981). Several studies have shown that patients with cancer tend to have low blood levels of retinol (Atukorala et al. 1979) but this might simply reflect the effect of nutritional deficiency on the synthesis of retinol binding protein (Tyler 1984). The reports in three large studies that patients with low blood retinol levels were associated with increased risk of subsequently developing cancer are exciting (Wald et al. 1980; Kark et al. 1981) but a third study failed to confirm this finding (Willet et al. 1984). High doses of retinol are extremely toxic but there is a possibility that synthetic retinoids might be of use in the treatment of cancer (Sporn & Newton 1979; Lancet 1980). β carotene has the advantage that unlike retinol it is not toxic and there are theoretical reasons for thinking it might be more effective in preventing malignancy (Peto et al. 1981). Further studies of this subject must be awaited with interest.

The possible actions of other vitamins in preventing cancer are discussed by Willet & MacMahon (1984).

11 Interaction of Drugs and Nutrition in the Elderly

Professor J.W.T. Dickerson

INTRODUCTION

One consequence of the high frequency of disease in the elderly is that they are given twice as many prescriptions as the national average (Royal College of Physicians 1984) and consume far more drugs than the young. It is not surprising therefore that adverse reactions are common in the elderly (Hurwitz 1969) and contribute to some 10% of admissions to geriatric units in hospitals (Williamson & Chaplin 1980). Age related changes in drug metabolism and elimination possibly exacerbated by nutritional deficiency predispose the elderly to drug related disease. The ingestion of multiple drugs increases the possibility of drug-drug interactions and failure to understand or follow instructions on how the drugs should be taken compounds the problem. A recent study in a teaching hospital also highlights the importance of prescribing errors as a cause of drug induced morbidity (Gosney & Tallis 1984).

This chapter is concerned with ways in which drugs may interact with food and nutrients, particularly vitamins. An understanding of these interactions may well increase the effectiveness of drug therapy and reduce the risk of iatrogenic morbidity.

THE METABOLISM OF DRUGS

Drugs are metabolised by enzymatic processes which occur in two stages (Williams 1967). The first stage involves the conversion of non-polar drugs to polar derivatives by N-dealkylation, deamination, hydroxylation, oxidation or reduction. These Stage I reactions are carried out by the 'mixed function oxidase' (MFO) system of enzymes which also catalyse the hydrolysis of a number of endogenous compounds such as steroid hormones and fatty acids. The MFO system involves reduced nicotinamide adenine dinucleotide (NADPH) and cytochrome P-450 and is predominantly located in the endoplasmic reticulum of the liver but it is also present in other tissues such as the lung and small intestine. In the rat the activity of the MFO system and its inductive response decrease with age after maturity (Kato & Takanaka 1968).

The second stage in the metabolism of drugs involves conjugation of the polar compounds formed in Stage I with glucuronic acid, sulphate or glycine. The final stage of elimination or detoxification is the excretion of the conjugate in the urine or bile. Thus after absorption, the levels of active drug in the circulation depend on the activity of the enzyme systems involved in drug metabolism and on renal function. Nutritional status affects not only the amount of body fat and therefore the ability of the body to sequester fat soluble drugs, but also the activity of enzyme systems and the extent to which drugs are bound to protein. Malnutrition decreases the protein binding of the following drugs chloramphenicol, digoxin, phenylbutazone, salicylate, sulphadiazine, tetracycline, thiopentone and warfarin but does not change the protein binding of streptomycin and sulphafurazole (Cusack & Denham 1984). It must be remembered however that other factors, particularly smoking and previous exposure to drugs can increase the activity of the MFO system by induction.

Animal studies show that the activity of the hepatic MFO system is affected by a number of micronutrients including potassium, folate and ascorbic acid. The factors which may increase drug toxicity in the elderly are summarised in Figure 11.1. (Dickerson 1980).

The effects of ageing per se on the protein binding, volume of distribution, half-life and renal elimination of drugs have been summarised by Cusack and Denham (1984). The effects, as one would expect, are different for different drugs, some being increased, some decreased and some unaffected. There is, as yet, little evidence that a healthy elderly person will absorb drugs differently from a younger person.

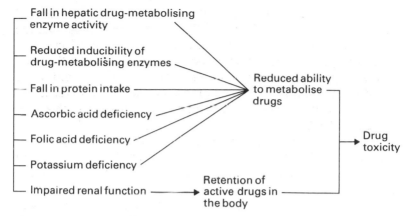

Fig. 11.1   Nutritional and other factors which may lead to increased drug toxicity in the elderly.

FOOD AND DRUG ABSORPTION

The influence of food on drug availability (Toothaker & Welling 1980), the absorption of antimicrobial agents (Welling & Tse 1982) and the absorption of other drugs in the elderly (Viswanathan & Welling 1984) have been extensively reviewed. Food may act as a barrier preventing drug access to the mucosal surface and depending on the chemical nature of the drug there is a possibility of interactions such as chelation with dietary constituents. Old people commonly take drugs at mealtimes because the meal acts as a convenient reminder and it is therefore important to consider possible effects of food on drug absorption.

Viswanathan & Welling (1984) have provided a list of anti-infective agents whose absorption is either reduced, delayed, unaffected or increased by food though the precise status of some agents remains uncertain. As a general rule most drugs are absorbed most rapidly in the fasting state. Mechanisms by which food might increase absorption of a drug such as griseofulvin include drug solubility in fatty foods, delayed gastric emptying and increased gastrointestinal secretion.

NUTRITIONAL CONSEQUENCES OF DRUGS COMMONLY GIVEN TO ELDERLY PATIENTS

The nutritional consequences of drugs taken for short periods of time by previously well nourished persons are unlikely to be of clinical significance. However in those elderly who are already susceptible to malnutrition a drug interaction may precipitate first a 'sub-clinical' vitamin deficiency with reduced blood and tissue levels, and subsequently, clinical deficiency disease (Figure 11.2). This sequence of changes becomes all the more likely when drugs are taken continuously over a long period of

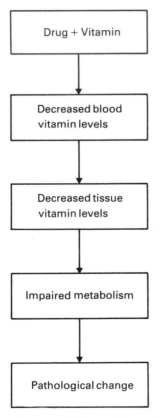

Fig. 11.2   Effect of drug vitamin interactions on vitamin status.

time. Some of the many drug nutrient interactions are listed in Table 11.1.

Table 11.1 Nutritional interaction of drugs commonly given to elderly patients (modified from Dickerson 1980).

Appetite
Depressed	Biguanides (e.g. phenformin & metformin)
	Digitalis
Increased	Sulphonylureas (e.g. tolbutamide, chlorpropamide glibenclamide)
	Phenothiazines (e.g. chlorpromazine)
	Benzodiazepines (e.g. diazepam; chlordiazepoxide)
	Anabolic agents (e.g. Durabolin)

Carbohydrate Metabolism
Hyperglycaemia	Thiazide diuretics; diazonide; corticosteroids; phenytoin
Hypoglycaemia	Sulphonylureas (when given with phenylbutazone, warfarin or dicoumarol)
	Alcohol, aspirin

Lipid Metabolism
Hyperlipidaemia	Chlorpromazine (cholesterol)
	Phenobarbitone (cholesterol & triglycerides)

Protein metabolism
Negative N Balance	Corticosteroids, tetracyclines

Mineral metabolism
Calcium depletion	Neomycin, colchicine
Hypocalcaemia	Frusemide; ethacrynic acid; phenolphthalein
Magnesium depletion	Thiazides; frusemide; ethacrynic acid; Gentamycin; cisplatin; neomycin; colchicine
Potassium depletion & Hypokalaemia	Thiazides; frusemide; ethacrynic acid; Phenolphthalein; corticosteroids; gentamycin
	Salicylates (Toxic dose); amphotericin B levodopa
Sodium depletion & Hyponatraemia	Thiazides; spironolactone; captopril; Chlorpropamide, tolbutamide, vincristine, Amitryptylene, mannitol
Iron deficiency	Aspirin, indomethacin
Zinc deficiency	Alcohol, penicillamine, digitalis

Table 11.1 — *cont'd*

Vitamins

Thiamin	Alcohol, antacids
Folic acid	Alcohol, anticonvulsants
Nicotinic acid	Isoniazid
Ascorbic acid	Aspirin, tetracyclines
Vitamin D	Anticonvulsants
Vitamin K	Purgatives, intestinal antibiotics

The phenomenon of drug vitamin interaction is well illustrated by the effects of anticonvulsant drugs, particularly phenytoin on folate and vitamin D status. Low serum folate levels are commonly found in patients taking anticonvulsants (Reynolds 1974) and occasional cases of megaloblastic anaemia due to folate deficiency have been reported. Anticonvulsants and other drugs such as the phenothiazines and tricyclics which induce the MFO system increase the requirement for folic acid which plays a role in the synthesis of cytochrome P-450. This may be the mechanism by which these drugs cause low blood levels of folate and deficiency if given for a sufficiently long-time to patients with inadequate intake of folate (Labadarios *et al.* 1978). It is not known to what extent anticonvulsant induced folic acid deficiency may exacerbate mental and neurological symptoms in these patients. However administration of folic acid may result in loss of control of epilepsy and it may be necessary to titrate drug dose against folate status in order to achieve the best clinical control with normal blood folate levels.

Long-term treatment with phenytoin or phenobarbital has been reported to cause osteomalacia (Dent *et al.* 1970). This effect has been attributed to induction of the MFO system by the anticonvulsant resulting in faster conversion of 25-hydroxycholecalciferol (25-HCC) to more polar inactive forms but this hypothesis has not been satisfactorally proved. An alternative mechanism is suggested by the observation that intestinal absorption of calcium may be low in patients taking anticonvulsants even though the serum 25-hydroxycholecalciferol level is normal (Wahl *et al.* 1981). Epileptic patients with osteomalacia may have normal plasma levels of 1,25-dihydroxycholecalciferol

Table 11.2 Adverse effects of 'Over the Counter' drugs used by the elderly.

Drugs	Indication for Prescription	Reasons for Self Medication	Adverse effects
Antacids	Hyperphosphataemia	Indigestion Flatulence 'Heart problems' Gas & bloating Gastric discomfort	Milk alkali syndrome Hypophosphataemia Sodium overload Magnesium overload Folate malabsorption Low thiamin status
	Recuce gastric pH		
Laxatives	Constipation Diseases of colon & rectum	Constipation Bowel obsession Intake of drugs that are constipating	Hypokalaemia Potassium deficiency Malabsorption of fat soluble vitamins (A, D & K) particularly due to mineral oil
Analgesics	Pain relief particularly for prevention of myocardial infarcts	Headache Insomnia Nervousness Hangover Cold & Cough Sore throat Pain	Iron deficiency anaemia due to gastric bleeding Folic acid deficiency Vitamin C deficiency

(1,25-di2HCC) even when levels of 25-oHCC are low (Jubiz *et al.* 1977). This suggests that the osteomalacia is unlikely to be due to defective renal production of the dihydroxy metabolite and supports the view that the anticonvulsant drug induces vitamin D resistance (Hahn *et al.* 1975). It seems uncertain whether anti- convulsants have a direct effect on intestinal calcium absorption or whether this is secondary to induced vitamin D deficiency (Corless *et al.* 1975) or to vitamin D resistance.

Although Ray and Rao (1974) found no evidence of hypocal- caemia in elderly patients who had been on anticonvulsants for periods from 6 weeks to 10 years, the possibility of precipitating deficiency in the elderly whose D status is already poor needs to be remembered.

Several other drug vitamin interactions are listed in Table 11.1.

Corticosteroids affect calcium metabolism in several ways including impairment of calcium absorption, mobilisation of calcium from the skeleton and hypercalciuria. They may also modify vitamin D metabolism as reduced levels of 1,25-dioHCC have been reported in children receiving glucocorticoids (Chesney *et al.* 1978).

Alcohol has many roles in society but in our present context must be considered as a drug and one which is consumed in sub- stantial amounts by some old people. As shown in Table 11.1 it interacts with thiamin and folic acid. A small proportion of alcoholics develop Wernicke's encephalopathy (see Chapter 6). Low blood folate levels are also common in all alcoholics but the risk is greater in spirit drinkers than beer drinkers since some kinds of beer are a good source of folate (Wu *et al.* 1975). The macrocytosis associated with alcohol is not due to folate defi- ciency but is a toxic effect and only rectified when the subjects cease drinking alcohol.

Many drugs given to the elderly lead to low blood levels of minerals (Table 11.1) either as a result of increased plasma volume or as a result of true depletion. Anaemia, iron deficiency and the probability that they may be due to gastrointestinal bleeding induced by various drugs were discussed in chapter 3. The possibility of zinc deficiency due to chelating drugs, such as penicillamine, occasionally used in the treatment of rheumatoid arthritis also needs to be remembered.

SELF MEDICATION

A number of drugs are readily available over the counter in Chemist shops and can be bought by the elderly or any other age group. Roe (1984) commented that up to 60% of the drugs consumed by elderly people may be obtained in this way. The drugs most commonly obtained without prescription (antacids, laxatives and analgesics) can also be prescribed but are usually taken by old people for the relief of rather vague symptoms (Table 11.2). The nutritional side-effects of these drugs may compound the problems caused by underlying disease, malnutrition and other drugs. Thus an elderly person with ischaemic heart disease already taking thiazide diuretics and digoxin who then takes laxatives may precipitate hypokalaemia and cardiac arrythmias.

Aspirin is another drug consumed in large doses which may be obtained with or without prescription. This drug interferes with intestinal absorption of vitamin C and entry of vitamin C into leucocytes (Basu 1981) and could exacerbate the tendency for old people to become vitamin C deficient or even develop clinical scurvy.

INTERACTIONS OF VITAMINS WITH DRUGS

Occasionally vitamin supplements may interfere with the actions of other drugs. The effect of folate supplements on anticonvulsant therapy was mentioned in an earlier section. Large doses of vitamin E may cause haemorrhage in patients receiving warfarin (Corrigan & Marcus 1974) while vitamin K will neutralise the effect of anticoagulant therapy.

CONCLUSIONS

The high frequency of disease in the elderly and the large numbers of drugs they consume mean that they are at very high risk of all types of adverse drug reactions including drug nutrient interactions. Physicians caring for the elderly should consider the possibility that the drugs they prescribe may interact with nutrients and exacerbate the risk of iatrogenic disease. The possibility that over the counter medications may also have a similar effect must also be borne in mind.

12 The Prevention of Vitamin Deficiency in the Elderly

J.R. Kemm

INTRODUCTION

Many of the ills of old age cannot be prevented but this is not true of vitamin deficiency which could be combatted by a policy of primary and secondary prevention. Secondary prevention involves early detection and correction of vitamin deficiencies before they cause symptoms or impair the quality of life. Primary prevention describes measures intended to stop vitamin deficiency from occuring at all. Successful primary prevention must not be restricted to measures directly affecting nutrient consumption but it must tackle all the intermediate causes (Figure 12.1) which lead indirectly to vitamin deficiency states in the elderly.

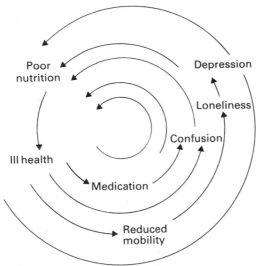

Fig. 12.1 Vicious circles of malnutrition.
The interaction of health and nutritional status.

INTERMEDIATE CAUSES

Poor Health

Healthy happy old people have adequate nutrient intakes and when vitamin deficiency is found in the elderly one must look at the whole quality of life, and not just at food consumption. Poor health is probably an aspect of old age which the elderly dislike most (Hunt 1978) and it may cause vitamin deficiency, not only by increasing vitamin requirements as described in Chapter 2, but also by interfering with the ability of the elderly to feed themselves.

Sixteen percent of men and 22% of women aged 85 or more were housebound and a further 64% of men and 53% of women had some handicapping illness or disability. Twenty seven percent of this age group were unable to cook a main meal, 13% were unable even to make a cup of tea and of those who were not housebound, less than half (46%) could do any shopping (Hunt 1978). More effective treatment of the many illnesses which limit the mobility of the elderly would improve not only their quality of life but also their nutritional status. Brocklehurst et al. (1978a) have stressed how frequently untreated but treatable conditions are found in the elderly. Foot problems deserve special mention as a very common cause of limited mobility which might be prevented by better chiropody services.

Dementia is one illness that may render an elderly person unable to plan and prepare adequate meals. The number of mentally infirm elderly is large and rising (British Medical Journal 1978) though estimates of prevalence vary from 10% (Kay et al. 1964) to 1.6% (Clarke et al. 1984). The relation between dementia and nutrition is discussed in Chapter 9 but there can be no doubt that the elderly mentally infirm are a group at risk of malnutrition and vitamin deficiency.

The increasing prevalence of disease with ageing is also accompanied by changes which, while they may be regarded as physiological still affect the nutrition of the elderly. Taste sensitivity (Bourliere et al. 1958; Grzegorezyk et al. 1979; Baker et al. 1983) and smell sensitivity (Schiffman & Pasternak 1979) decline with age and will impair the ability of the elderly to enjoy food. Little can be done to restore taste acuity though improved oral hygiene might have a small effect (Langar & Yearlich 1976) but those who cater for the elderly must bear in mind the need to stimulate dimmed taste sensation.

Poor dentition is another common problem in the elderly. Seventy two percent of the elderly are edentulous and of these only 30% have satisfactory false dentition (Todd & Walker 1980) Difficulties with teeth easily restrict the range of foods eaten and though there is no clear association between bad dentition and malnutrition (DHSS 1972; Elwood & Bates 1972), it still seems probable that correcting inadequate dentures would improve the ability of the elderly to feed themselves adequately.

Loneliness and Isolation

After ill health loneliness was the most frequent complaint of the elderly, while the company of family and friends was the thing which the elderly mentioned as being enjoyed most often (Hunt 1978). A high proportion of the elderly live alone and feel lonely. Hunt (1978) found that 5% of those aged over 75 had no living relatives, 45% received visits from relatives and friends less than once a week and 29% reported receiving no visitors at all. In another survey of a country town 23% of those aged over 75 were classified as isolated (Clarke *et al.* 1984).

Eating is very much a social activity and the giving and receiving of affection are commonly associated with the giving and receiving of food. An elderly person is much more likely to spend time and trouble preparing a meal which is eaten with company than in preparing a meal for themselves alone. Attempts to increase food consumption without considering the associated isolation are unlikely to be effective.

Inevitably old age is a time when one loses friends and contemporaries but there are many interventions which might reduce the feeling of loneliness. Promotion of social and special interest clubs help to reduce isolation, but unless transport is also provided they may be ineffective because the elderly are unable to get to them. Equally important are visitors at home such as relatives, volunteer visitors, good neighbours and ministers of religion, all of whom help to reduce isolation. Tradesmen who call at the house such as the postman and milkman are valuable not only for the services which they provide but also as links with the community. Any intervention designed to decrease loneliness in the elderly can be expected incidentally to improve nutritional status.

Ignorance of elementary homecraft is often cited as a cause of malnutrition in the elderly and 'bachelor' scurvy is a well recognised condition. Elderly widowers whose food has always been prepared for them first by their mothers and then by their wives may find it difficult to learn the skills of catering for themselves in later life, but sympathetic advice is usually adequate to correct this situation.

Improving nutrition and quality of life at home is usually the best way of preventing vitamin deficiency in the elderly. However there are a very few old people who find living in their own homes too difficult and too lonely for whom a move into residential accommodation where food, company and care are provided may be the best way of improving nutritional status and enjoyment of life.

Poverty

The elderly frequently have less material wealth and less disposable income than their younger neighbours. This difference in disposable income is reflected in expenditure. When the non-retired person living alone spent £13.59 on food, £4.00 on alcoholic drinks, £4.99 on fuel light and power, £5.84 on clothes and £5.86 on consumer durables, the retired person mainly dependent upon a state pension and living alone spent £9.99 on food, £0.56 on alcoholic drinks, £4.78 on fuel, light and power, £1.69 on clothes and £1.20 on consumer durables ([Table 10] Department of Employment 1982). Comparisons of other household types tell the same story, the retired elderly and especially those relying on a pension for their income, spend less on food and less on clothes.

Real shortage of money may be compounded by difficulty in managing what money they have. The elderly remember days when chocolate bars cost one old penny (0.42p) and frequently find it difficult to adjust to modern prices. Their parents were terrified of ending their days in the workhouse (institutions for the destitute) and fears like these may make the elderly reluctant to spend what little income they have.

Changing retail patterns have also put the elderly at a disadvantage. Supermarkets, hypermarkets and bulk buying have all helped to keep down the retail price of food, but their growth has been accompanied by a decline of small local traders. The elderly lacking mobility and access to transport have frequently been unable to take advantage of these developments. Bulk buying is also difficult for those who cannot carry large shopping bags and who do not have readily available cash reserves. The elderly often have to buy small quantities from local traders and consequently get less nutrients for each pound expended.

Discussion of cause immediately suggest methods of prevention. The most economically vulnerable group are those who are forced to rely on their pension. Increases in pension would be expected to increase expenditure on food and fuel. Other ways of directing resources to the elderly such as fuel and housing rebates would also be expected to increase expenditure on food. Trends in retailing cannot be reversed but the elderly might be enabled to share the benefits of new developments by measures such as community bus services which give them access to the supermarkets.

HYPOTHERMIA

There is a parallel to be drawn between hypothermia and vitamin deficiency in the elderly. While overt hypothermia (body temperature $< 35\,^{\circ}$C) is not often recognised, low body temperatures ($< 35.5\,^{\circ}$C) are very common, being found in 10% of the elderly (Fox *et al.* 1973). The underlying causes of hypothermia and nutritional deficiency are the same, namely a malign combination of ill health, poor living conditions, financial constraints and impaired homeostatic systems. Those who become hypothermic tend to have low food intakes (Bastow, Rawlings & Allison 1983a) and it is possible that those with thiamin deficiency might be at an especially high risk of hypothermia (Phillip & Smith 1973). Hypothermia and vitamin deficiency in the elderly can both be regarded as manifestations of the same underlying problems.

SPECIFIC INTERVENTIONS

Meals on Wheels

The provision of meals at home (Meals on Wheels) in the UK was pioneered by voluntary bodies during the 1939–45 war. Subsequently the responsibility for providing these services was placed on the local authorities but they still often use voluntary bodies as agents for discharging this responsibility. The service has been expanded progressively until a few years ago (Figure 12.2).

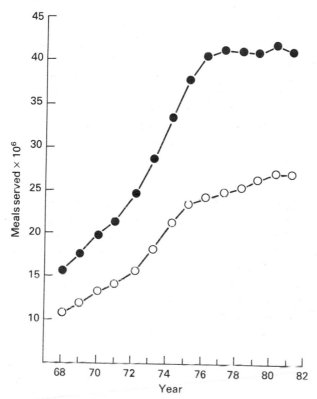

Fig. 12.2 Growth of local authority meals services.
The number of meals served at the clients home in a year (O——O) and the total number of meals served (●——●) are shown. Before 1972 the figures are for the year ending 31st December and after 1972 for the year ending 31st March. (Source: Health and Personal Social Services Statistics DHSS).

The explicitly stated objective of the meals on wheels service is to 'provide a nutritional mid-day meal for people who are temporarily or permanently incapable of doing so for themselves'. More important, however, are two unstated objectives implicit in the actions and caring attitudes of those who provide the service. One is a nutritional objective of preventing nutritional deficiency in elderly people by supplementing the dietary intake of those in whom it might otherwise be deficient. The other is a non-nutritional objective of providing social contact and unobtrusive surveillance for the housebound elderly (Kemm 1979; Goldberg & Connelly 1982). The service might be more effective if these objectives had been explicitly stated.

Evaluating the direct effect on nutrition of Meals on Wheels is difficult, but one study in Portsmouth suggested that the vitamin C and protein content were often low and that problems of portion control resulted in widely varying intakes of nutrients (Davies 1981). It is particularly difficult to maintain the vitamin C content of a meal which is kept hot before serving. Newer industrial catering methods enable prepared meals to be heated by microwave immediately before delivery to the client or heated by the client himself (Armstrong 1981).

Obviously uneaten meals do not improve nutritional status and it is therefore important that meals look attractive and are palatable. Delivered meals should also supplement nutrient intake and not simply replace other meals. The Portsmouth study (Davies 1981) found that dietary intakes of most clients were increased on Meals on Wheels day's but another study from Sheffield suggested that delivered meals might displace more nutritious food (Booth 1977).

If Meals on Wheels are to have a significant effect on nutritional status of the elderly they must either be delivered most days of the week, or else be fortified with several days requirements of certain nutrients such as vitamins. The majority of Meals on Wheels clients receive only one or two meals a week and the meals are not fortified.

The foregoing discussion suggests that the direct contribution of Meals on Wheels to nutritional status is small. What of the second implicit objective? Are they effective in reducing isolation and thereby improving nutritional status? Do they 'bring to the old people not only a meal which they may be unable to cook for themselves but also friendliness' (Goldberg & Connelly 1982). Many clients may value the friendliness more highly than the meal (Kemm 1981). The constraints imposed by the nutritional objective make it difficult to meet the non nutritional objectives. A typical 'meals' round seeks to deliver hot meals to 20 or more clients between 12.00 and 14.00 hours allowing a mean time of six minutes inclusive of journey time for each client. Concentration on mealtime also makes it difficult to recruit volunteer helpers since many who would gladly help at other times have home commitments at lunch hour.

Lunch Clubs and Day Centres

Like Meals on Wheels, lunch clubs have two implicit objectives, firstly as a nutritional objective of supplementing nutrient intake and secondly as a non nutritional objective of providing social contact. Unlike Meals on Wheels these two objectives are readily compatible and complement each other. The formidable difficulties and expense of distributing a hot meal to several widely spaced houses are avoided and it is relatively easy to provide a hot nutritious meal on one site. Attractive presentation of food on the plate is easy and the social surroundings promote a good appetite. Lunch clubs can easily be combined with day centres and social clubs.

The main restriction on lunch clubs is the difficulty many elderly have in reaching them but the cost of bringing the meal to the elderly may not be much less than the cost of bringing the elderly to the meal. Also lunch clubs cannot meet the needs of the sizeable minority of elderly who would benefit from some increased nutrient intake but dislike the ambience of clubs and social centres.

CATERING IN INSTITUTIONS

In theory when an old person enters residential care there ought to be no further worries about his nutrient intake. Twenty years ago it was recognised that there were problems with the quality of food in some institutions (Platt 1963) and food hygiene (Lancet 1980) and food nutritional value (Evans 1978) continue to cause problems. Vitamin C is all too easily destroyed by over-cooking food and is a particular problem in institutional catering (see Chapter 9). Constant attention to the palatability and nutrient content of food in hospitals and residential homes is necessary to prevent vitamin deficiency in their elderly residents.

TOXICITY

Before considering fortification and supplementation with vitamins we must be satisfied that there is no significant risk of adverse effects.

The toxicity of vitamin A is well recognised and there are numerous reports of severe illness or death due to ingestion of excessive amounts of vitamin A (Muentner et al. 1971). The clinical features of vitamin A toxicity include anorexia, irritability, headache, itchy skin, hair loss, exfoliative dermatitis, raised intracranial pressure and convulsions.

Vitamin D is also toxic in excess causing hypercalcaemia, ectopic calcification, renal failure and convulsions and there are several reports of vitamin D poisoning (Paterson 1980). The wide individual variation in vitamin D requirement and threshold for toxicity is particularly worrying and it is possible that one man's requirement is another man's toxic dose (See chapter 5). Toxicity can be avoided by checking serum calcium at intervals in those for whom vitamin D is prescribed.

The toxic effects of water soluble vitamins have recently been reviewed by Alhadeff et al. (1984) but generally they only occur with extraordinarily high intakes and are unimportant. High doses of nicotinic acid cause peripheral vasodilatation and facial flushing, but this is an acute and self limiting problem. Pyridoxine has caused sensory neuropathy with axonal degeneration when given in huge doses (Schaumberg et al. 1983).

There has been much discussion over the safety of megadose vitamin C therapy. Diarrhoea is an occasional but not a serious problem. There have also been isolated reports of oxalate renal stones and increased requirement for vitamin C resulting in scurvy when megadosage was suddenly stopped. There is little doubt that in most people megadosage is harmless (Hughes 1982), but the possibility of serious side-effects in a few people with idiosyncratic vitamin C metabolism cannot be ruled out.

Folate is probably not toxic but the possibility of precipitating subacute combined degeneration in those who are vitamin B_{12} deficient (see Chapter 3) must be borne in mind.

Interaction of vitamin supplements with drugs has been discussed in Chapter 11.

FORTIFICATION

Certain foods such as bread (nicotinic acid and riboflavin), margarine (vitamins A and D) are nearly always fortified while others such as fruit juices (vitamin C) and breakfast cereal (multiple vitamins) are frequently fortified.

Technically it would be possible to fortify foods for the elderly but there are practical and ethical objections. The elderly eat the same foods as younger members of the population and it would be difficult to identify for fortification foods eaten predominantly by the elderly. Experience with fortification of infant milks with vitamin D (Cohen 1957) suggests that fortification even to low levels might expose some individuals to the risk of vitamin D toxicity since there would be wide variation both in intakes of fortified foods and in susceptibility to toxic effects. Some may also view fortification as involuntary medication and object to it on ethical grounds.

Fortification in most circumstances is neither an acceptable nor an effective way of preventing vitamin deficiency in the elderly. It may have a limited role in institutional catering.

SUPPLEMENTATION

Low blood vitamin levels can easily be restored to normal by taking vitamin supplements provided that a large enough dose is used (Griffiths et al. 1967; Brocklehurst et al. 1968; Burr et al. 1975; MacLennan & Hamilton 1977b; Corless et al. 1978; Bates et al. 1979; Schorah et al. 1979; Vir & Love 1979; Baker et al. 1980; Johnson et al. 1980).

Distributing supplements to all elderly persons would be an expensive and difficult task, but ensuring that they were consumed would be virtually impossible. The problems of compliance with drug therapy in the elderly are well recognised (Royal College of Physicians 1984). Most geriatricians are attempting to reduce the numbers of medication being taken and addition of a multivitamin capsule could well increase confusion over medication. The groups most at risk of vitamin deficiency namely those living alone and the mentally infirm are the groups least likely to take supplements. Mass distribution of vitamin supplements would probably not be an effective way of preventing vitamin deficiency in the elderly. Mass supplementation also has the disadvantage that it is solely a nutritional intervention and does not tackle any of the underlying causes of vitamin deficiency. Nutrients in pills do not give the social and personal pleasures associated with eating.

On the other hand carefully supervised vitamin supplementation is very useful as part of the care of individual elderly patients known to be at risk of deficiency.

Vitamin supplements may be obtained either on prescription or over the counter. At the moment very few elderly people in the UK take vitamin supplements. One survey found that 5% of elderly men and 6.5% of elderly women took supplements (DHSS 1979a) and another found that 4% of men and 8% of women aged over 75 took supplements (OPCS 1973). In the USA many more elderly people take supplements (56% in one survey (Garry et al. 1982)).

NON NUTRITIONAL INTERVENTIONS

A host of other services may indirectly influence the nutritional status of the elderly. Local authorities provide home helps to assist with personal and domestic tasks for those who are unable to do these for themselves. Only a small part of the home help's time is devoted to tasks directly relevant to nutrition such as preparing meals and shopping (shopping 10%, preparing meals 7% in one survey (Howell et al. 1979) and the majority of their time is spent on other tasks such as cleaning and washing. However home helps probably make a major indirect contribution to the nutritional status of their clients by improving morale and preventing isolation.

The vast majority of frail elderly who need care and attention receive it not from health and social services but from their friends and relatives (especially spouses and daughters). The activities of these informal carers make a major contribution to preventing vitamin deficiency in the elderly. They provide food and care for their charges in a way that the statutory services could not replace. Belatedly their major contribution is being recognised and measures designed to support these informal carers must be seen as playing a crucial part in the prevention of nutritional deficiency.

SECONDARY PREVENTION

A policy of primary prevention needs to be supported by a secondary prevention programme. The possibility of vitamin deficiency should always be borne in mind by all those who care for the elderly. Hospital staff, GP's and the primary care team, home helps and social workers ought to be ready to suspect inadequate nutrition.

Much of this book has been concerned with the difficulties of defining and diagnosing vitamin deficiency but fortunately these difficulties need not hinder prevention. When vitamin deficiency is suspected, supplementation will rapidly correct the short-term nutritional deficiency and the underlying problems can then be tackled.

There are a few occasions when immediate supplementation is not appropriate. Where B_{12} deficiency is suspected the diagnosis needs to be established before giving supplements since treatment, if needed, should be lifelong. Similarly if it is essential to establish the diagnosis, all necessary blood samples must be taken before giving supplements. The problems of vitamin toxicity have been discussed earlier but only occur with prolonged high dosage and do not occur if the patient's supplementation is properly monitored.

Vitamin supplementation is generally safe and if an occasional patient who is not vitamin deficient receives vitamin supplements it does them no harm. It is better to err on the side of overdiagnosing vitamin deficiency states, than underdiagnosing them.

CONCLUSION

Those who make national policy should realise that vitamin deficiency in the elderly could largely be prevented if more resources were allocated to this group. The medical profession and others caring for the elderly should realise that vitamin deficiency still occurs, but if recognised can be easily corrected.

REFERENCES

Aaron J.F., Gallagher J.C., Anderson J., Stasiak L., Longton E.B., Nordin B.E.C. & Nicholson M. (1974) Frequency of osteomalacia and osteoporosis in fractures of proximal femur. *Lancet* **1**, 229-31.

Aitken J.M. (1984) Relevance of Osteoporosis in women with fracture neck of femur. *British Medical Journal* **288**, 597-601.

Aksoy M., Basu T.K., Brient J. & Dickerson J.W.T. (1980) Thiamin status of patients treated with drug combinations containing 5-fluorouracil. *European Journal of Cancer* **16**, 1041-5.

Alfrey A.C., Miller N.L. & Butkus D. (1974) Evaluation of body magnesium stores. *Journal of Laboratory and Clinical Medicine* **84**, 153-62.

Algeri A., Consolazione A., Colderini G., Achilli G., Canas E.P. & Garattini S. (1979) Effect of administration of (d-Ala) methionine-enkephalin on the serotonin metabolism in rat brain. *Experimentia* **34**, 1488-9.

Alhadeff L., Gualtieri L.T. & Lipton M. (1984) Toxic effects of water soluble vitamins. *Nutrition Review* **42**, 33-40.

Allan R.J., DiMauro S., Coulter D.L., Papadimitriou A. & Rothenburg S.P. (1983) Kearns-Sayre syndrome with reduced plasma and cerebrospinal fluid folate. *Annals of Neurology* **13**, 679-82.

Alleyne G.A.O., Hay R.W., Picou D.I., Stanfield JP. & Whitehead R.G. (1977) *Protein Energy Malnutrition*. Arnold, London.

Anand M.P. (1964) Iatrogenic megaloblastic anaemia with neurological complications. *Scottish Medical Journal* **9**, 388-90.

Anderson B.B., Peart M.B. & Fulford-Jones E.E. (1970) The measurement of serum pyridoxal by a microbiological assay using Lactobacillus casei. *Journal of Clinical Pathology* **23**, 232-42.

Anderson I., Campbell A.E.R., Dunn A. & Runciman J.B.M. (1966) Osteomalacia in elderly women. *Scottish Medical Journal* **2**, 429-35.

Anderson T.W., Beaton G.H., Corey P.N. & Spero L. (1975) Winter illness and vitamin C: the effect of relatively low doses. *Canadian Medical Association Journal* **112**, 823-6.

Anderson W.F. & Cowan N.R. (1966) Hand grip pressure in older people. *British Journal of Preventative and Social Medicine* **20**, 141-7.

Andersson M., Walker A.R.P. & Falcke H.C. (1956) An investigation of the rarity of infantile scurvy among the South African Bantu. British Journal of Nutrition 10, 101–5.

Andrews J. & Brook M. (1966). Leucocyte-vitamin-C content and clinical signs in the elderly. Lancet 1, 1350–1.

Andrews, J., Brook M. & Allen M.A. (1966) Influence of abode and season on the vitamin C status of the elderly. Gerontologia Clinica 8, 257–66.

Andrews J., Letcher M., & Brook M. (1969) Vitamin C supplementation in the elderly: a 17 month trial in an old persons' home. British Medical Journal 2, 416–18.

Anthony H.M. & Schorah C.J. (1982) Severe hypovitaminosis C in lung cancer patients: the utilisation of vitamin C in surgical repair and lymphocyte related host resistance. British Journal of Cancer 46, 354–67.

Araya M., Silink S.J., Nobile S. & Walker-Smith J.A. (1975) Blood vitamin levels in children with gastroenteritis. Australian and New Zealand Journal of Medicine 51, 239–50.

Armstrong J. (1981) Meals on wheels a new approach. Hospital Equipment and Supplies: Catering Supplement 72–3.

Asplund K., Normonk M. & Patterson V. (1981) Nutritional assessment of psychogeriatric patients. Age and Ageing 10, 87–94.

Atukorala S., Basu T.K., Dickerson J.W.T., Donaldson D. & Sakula A. (1979) Vitamin A, zinc and lung cancer. British Journal of Cancer 40, 927–31.

Atukorala S., Dickerson J.W.T., Basu T.K. & McElwain T. (1982) Longitudinal studies of nutritional status in patients having chemotherapy for testicular teratomas. Clinical Oncology 9, 3–10.

Axelrod A.E., Carter B.B., McCoy R.H. & Geisinger R. (1947) Circulating antibodies in vitamin-deficiency states. I. Pyridoxine, riboflavin and pantothenic deficiencies. Proceedings of Society for Experimental Biology and Medicine 66, 137.

Axelrod A.E. & Trakatellis A.C. (1964) Induction of tolerance to skin homografts by administering splenic cells to pyridoxine-deficient mice. Proceedings for Society for Experimental Biology and Medicine 116, 206.

Axelrod A.E., Trakatellis A.C., Bloch II. & Stinebring W.R. (1963) Effect of pyridoxine deficiency upon delayed hypersensitivity in guinea pigs. Journal of Nutrition 79, 161–7.

Baird I.M., Hughes R.E., Wilson H.K., Davies J.E. & Howard A.N. (1979) The effects of ascorbic acid and flavinoids on the occurrence of symptoms normally associated with the common cold. American Journal of Clinical Nutrition 32, 1686–90.

168   *References*

168   *References*

168   *References*

168   *References*

168   *References*

Baker H., Frank O. & Jaslow S.P. (1980) Oral versus intramuscular vitamin supplementation for hypovitaminosis in the elderly. *Journal of American Geriatrics Society* **28**, 42–5.

Baker K.A., Didcock E.A., Kemm J.R. & Patrick J.M. (1983) Effect of age, sex and illness on salt taste detection threshold. *Age and Ageing* **12**, 159–65.

Baker M.R., McDonnell H., Peacock M. & Nordin B.E.C. (1979) Plasma 25-hydroxy vitamin D concentrations in patients with fractures of the femoral neck. *British Medical Journal* **1**, 589.

Ballag W. (1983) Vitamin A and retinoids: from nutrition to pharmacotherapy in dermatology and oncology. *Lancet* **1**, 860–2.

Bamji M.S. (1969) Glutathione reductase activity in red blood cells and riboflavin nutritional status in humans. *Clinica Chimica Acta* **26**, 263–9.

Bang B.G., Bang F.B. & Foard M.A. (1972) Lymphocyte depression induced in chickens on diets deficient in vitamin A and other components. *American Journal of Pathology* **68**, 147.

Bannerjee A.K., Lane P J & Meichen F.W. (1978) Vitamin C and osteoporosis in old age. *Age and Ageing* **7**, 16–18.

Banos G., Daniel P.M. & Pratt O.E. (1971) Inhibition of entry of L-arginine into the brain of the rat, *in vivo*, by L-lysine or L-ornithine. *Journal of Physiology* **214**, 24–5p.

Banos G., Daniel P.M. & Pratt O.E. (1974) Saturation of a shared mechanism which transports L-arginine and L-lysine into the brain of the living rat. *Journal of Physiology* **236**, 29–41.

Banos G., Daniel P.M. & Pratt O.E. (1978) The effect of age upon the entry of some amino acids into the brain and their incorporation into cerebral protein. *Developmental Medicine and Child Neurology* **20**, 335–46.

Barber T.L., Nockels C.F. & Jochim M.M. (1977) Vitamin E enhancement of Venezuelan equine encephalomyelitis antibody response in guinea pigs. *American Journal of Veterinary Research* **38**, 731–4.

Barker B.M. (1982) Vitamin A. In Barker B.M. & Bender D.A. (eds) *Vitamins in Medicine* **2**, 211–90. Heinemann, London.

Barker B.M. & Bender D.A. (1980) *Vitamins in Medicine* **1** and **2**. Heinemann, London.

Barragry J.M., France M.W., Corless D., Gupta S.P., Swilala S., Boucher B.J. & Cotton R.D. (1978) Cholecalciferol absorption in the elderly. *Clinical Science and Molecular Medicine* **54**, 28.

Bartley W., Krebs H.A. & O'Brien J.R.P. (1953) Vitamin C requirement of human adults. *Medical Research Council Special Reports Series* **280** HMSO, London.

Bartus R.T., Dean R.L., Sherman K.A., Friedman F. and Beer B. (1982)

Profound effects of combining choline and piracetam on memory enhancement and cholinergic function in aged rats. *Neurobiology of Ageing* **2**, 105–11.

Bastow M.D., Rawlings J. & Allison S.P. (1983a) Undernutrition, hypothermia and injury in elderly women with fractured femur; an injury response to altered metabolism. *Lancet* **1**, 143–6.

Bastow M.D., Rawlings J. & Allison S.P. (1983b) Benefits of supplementary tube feeding after fractured neck of femur: a randomised controlled trial. *British Medical Journal* **287**, 1589–92.

Basu T.K. (1981) The influence of drugs with particular reference to effect of aspirin on bioavailibility of vitamin C. In Counsell J.N. & Hornig D.H. (eds) *Vitamin C* 273–81. Applied Science Publishers, London.

Basu T.K., Aksoy M. & Dickerson J.W. (1979) Effects of 5-Fluorouracil on the thiamine status of adult female rats. *Chemotherapy* **25**, 70–6.

Basu T.K., Raven R.W., Dickerson J.W.T. & Williams D.C. (1974) Leucocyte ascorbic acid and urinary hydroxyproline levels in patients bearing breast tumour with skeletal metastases. *European Journal of Cancer* **10**, 507–11.

Basu T.K., Smethurst M., Gillett M.B., Donaldson D., Jordan S.J., Williams D.C. & Hicklin J.A. (1978) Ascorbic acid therapy for the relief of bone pain in Paget's disease. *Acta Vitaminologica Enzymologica* (Milano) **32**, 45–9.

Batata M., Spray G.H., Bolton F.G., Higgins C.H. & Wolner L. (1967) Blood and bone marrow changes in elderly patients with special reference to folic acid, vitamin B_{12}, iron and ascorbic acid. *British Medical Journal* **2**, 667–9.

Bates C.J., Black A.E., Phillips D.R., Wright A.J.A. & Southgate D.A.T. (1982) The discrepancy between normal folate intakes and the folate RDA. *Human Nutrition* **36A**, 422–39.

Bates C.J., Fleming M., Paul A.A., Black A.E. & Mander A.R. (1980) Folate status and its relation to vitamin C in healthy elderly men and women. *Age and Ageing* **9**, 241–8.

Bates C.J., Prentice A.M., Paul A.A., Sutcliffe B.A., Watkinson M. & Whitehead R.G. (1981) Riboflavin status in Gambian pregnant and lactating women and its implications for recommended dietary allowances. *American Journal of Clinical Nutrition* **34**, 928–35.

Bates C.J., Rutishauer I.H.E., Black A.E., Paul A.A., Mandal A.R. & Patnaik B.K. (1979) Long-term vitamin status and dietary intake of healthy subjects to vitamin C. *British Journal of Nutrition* **42**, 43–56.

Bayoumi R.A. & Rosalki S.E. (1976) Evaluation of methods of coenzyme activation of erythrocyte enzymes for detection of deficiency of vitamins B_1, B_2 and B_6. *Clinical Chemistry* **22**, 327–35.

Beisel W.R., Edelman R., Nauss K. & Suskind R.M. (1981) Single nutrient effects on immunological functions. *Journal of America Medical Association* **254**, 53–8.

Bender D.A. (1980) Niacin. In Barker B.M. & Bender D.A. (eds) *Vitamins in Medicine* 1, 315–47. Heinemann, London.

Bender D.A. (1982) Vitamin C. In Barker B.M. & Bender D.A. (eds) *Vitamins in Medicine* 2, 1–68. Heinemann, London.

Bender D.A., Early C.J. & Lees A.J. (1979) Niacin depletion in Parkinsonian patients treated with l-dopa, benserazide and carbidopa. *Clinical Science* **56**, 89–93.

Bender D.A. & Smith W.R.D. (1978) Inhibition of kynurenine hydrolase by benserazide, carbidopa and other aromatic hydrazine derivatives: evidence for subclinical iatrogenic niacin deficiency. *Biochemical Society Transactions* **6**, 120–2.

Bernstein D.S., Sadowsky N., Hezsted D.M., Guri C.D. & Stare F.J. (1966) Prevalence of osteoporosis in high and low fluoride areas in North Dakota. *Journal of the American Medical Association* **198**, 499–504.

Berry W.T.C. (1968) Protein status in the elderly. *Proceedings of the Nutrition Society* **27**, 185–96.

Beutler E. (1969) Effect of flavin compounds on glutathione reductase activity: *in vivo* and *in vitro* studies. *Journal of Clinical Investigation* **48**, 1957–66.

Bhatt H., Daniel P.M., Linnell J.C., Love E.R. & Pratt O.E. (1980) The influx of cyancobalamin into the brain of the rat, *in vivo*. *Journal of Physiology* **308**, 88p.

Black A.E., Ashby D.R., Day K.C., Bates C.J. & Paul A.A. (1983) Analytical versus food table values for vitamin C in foods: the effect on calculated vitamin C intake of elderly subjects. *Human Nutrition: Applied Nutrition* **37A**, 9–22.

Blass J.P. & Gibson G.E. (1977) Abnormality of a thiamine-requiring enzyme in Wernicke-Korsakoff syndrome. *New England Journal of Medicine* **297**, 1367–70.

Blass J.P., Piacentini S., Boldiszar E. & Baker A. (1982) Kinetic studies of mouse brain transketolase. *Journal of Neurochemistry* **39**, 729–33.

Blessed G. (1980). In P.J. Roberts (ed.) Biochemistry of Dementia. Wiley, Chichester.

Bodor N. & Simpkins J.W. (1983) Redox delivery system for specific sustained release of dopamine. *Science* **221**, 65–7.

Booth T. (1977) Nutrition survey strikes a warning note for the elderly. *Health and Social Services Journal* **77**, 1050–1.

Bourliere F. Cendron H. & Rapaport A. (1958) Modification avec l'age de seuils gustatifs de perception et de reconnaissance aux saveurs salee et sucree chez l'homme. *Gerontologia* **2**, 104–12.

Bowen D.M. & Davison A.N. (1984) Dementia in the elderly: Biochemical aspects. *Journal of the Royal College of Physicians*, London, **18**, 25-7.

Bowers E.F. & Kubic M.M. (1965) Vitamin C levels in old people and their response to ascorbic acid and to the juice of acerola. *British Journal of Clinical Practice* **19**, 141-7.

Brennan M.F. (1981) Total parenteral nutrition in the management of the cancer patient. *Acta Chirugica Scandinavica Supplement* **507**, 428-34.

Briggs M. & Briggs M. (1972) Vitamin C requirements and oral contraceptives. *Nature* **238**, 277.

Brin M. (1962) Erythrocyte transketolase in early thiamin deficiency *Annals of New York Academy of Sciences* **98**, 528-41.

Brin, M. (1964) Erythrocyte as a biopsy tissue for functional evaluation of thiamine adequacy. *Journal of American Medical Association* **187**, 762-9.

Brin M., Tai M., Ostashever A.S. & Kalinsky H. (1960) Effects of thiamine deficiency on activity of erythrocyte transketolase. *Journal of Nutrition* **71**, 273-81.

British Medical Journal Leading Article (1979) Wernicke's encephalopathy. *British Medical Journal* **2**, 291-2.

British Medical Journal Leading Article (1978) The quiet epidemic. *British Medical Journal* **1**, 1.

Brocklehurst J.C. (1975) Ageing in the autonomic nervous system. *Age and Ageing* **4**, Suppl. 7-17.

Brocklehurst J.C., Carty M.H., Leeming J.T. & Robinson J.M. (1978a) Medical screening of old people accepted for residential care. *Lancet* **2**, 141-2.

Brocklehurst J.C., Exton-Smith A.N., Lempert Barber S.M., Hunt L.P. & Palmer M.K. (1978b) Fracture of the femur in old age: a two-centre study of associated clinical factors and the cause of the fall. *Age and Ageing* **7**, 7-15.

Brocklehurst J.C., Griffiths L.L., Taylor G.F., Marks J., Scott D.L. & Blackley J. (1968) The clinical features of chronic vitamin deficiency: A therapeutic trial in geriatric hospital patients. *Gerontologia Clinica* **10**, 309-20.

Brown J.R.F., Bakouska A. & Millard P.H. (1976) Vitamin D status of patients with femoral neck fractures. *Age and Ageing* **5**, 127-31.

Burgert S.L. & Anderson C.F. (1979) An evaluation of upper arm measurements used in nutritional assessment. *American Journal of Clinical Nutrition* **32**, 2136-142.

Burke B.S. (1947) The dietary history as a research tool. *Journal of the American Dietetic Association* **23**, 1041-6.

Burr M.L., Elwood P.C., Hole D.V., Hurley R.J. & Hughes R.E. (1974a)

Plasma and leucocyte ascorbic acid levels in the elderly. American Journal of Clinical Nutrition 27, 144–51.

Burr M.L., Hurley R.J. & Sweetnam P.M. (1975) Vitamin C supplementation of old people with low blood levels. Gerontologia Clinica 17, 236–43.

Burr M.L., Lennings C.I. & Milbank J.E. (1982a) The prognostic significance of weight and of vitamin C status in the elderly. Age and Ageing 11, 249–55.

Burr M.L., Milbank J.E. & Gibbs D. (1982b) The nutritional status of the elderly. Age and Ageing 11, 89–96.

Burr M.L. & Phillips K.M. (1984) Anthropometric norms in the elderly: British Journal of Nutrition 51, 165–9.

Burr M.L., Sweetnam P.M., Hurley R.J. & Powell G.H. (1974b) Effects of age and intake on plasma ascorbic acid levels. Lancet 1, 163–4.

Busher G.L., Lockwood T.J., Cochrane H.R., Delves H.T. & Hall M.R.P. (1982) Serum zinc in old age. Journal of Clinical and Experimental Gerontology 4, 249–56.

Butterworth R.F. (1982) Neurotransmitter function in thiamine-deficiency neuropathy. Neurochemistry International 4, 449–664.

Buttery J.E., Milner C.R. & Chamberlain B.R. (1980) Correction for the suppressive effect of haemoglobin on NADH absorbance in the transketolase assay. Clinica Chimica Acta 102, 221–5.

Buzby G.P., Mullen J.L., Stein T.P., Miller E.E., Hobbs C.L. & Rosato E.F. (1980) Host tumour interaction and nutrient supply. Cancer 45, 2940–8.

Calman K.C. (1982) Cancer cachexia. British Journal of Hospital Medicine 27, 23–34.

Cameron E. & Pauling L. (1974) The orthomolecular treatment of cancer. I. The role of ascorbic acid in host resistance. Chemico Biological Interactions 9, 273.

Cameron E. & Pauling L. (1978) Supplemental ascorbate in the supportive treatment of cancer: Re-evaluation of prolongation of survival times in terminal human cancer. Proceedings of the National Academy of Sciences USA 75, 4538–42.

Campbell G., Kemm J.R., Hosking D. & Boyd R.V. (1984) How common is osteomalacia in the elderly? Lancet 2, 386–8.

Campbell P.A., Cooper H.R., Heinzerling R.H. & Tengerdy R.P. (1974) Vitamin E enhances in vitro immune response by normal and non-adherent spleen cells. Proceedings of Society for Experimental Biology and Medicine 146, 465–9.

Carleen M.H., Weissman N. & Ferrebee J.W. (1944) Subclinical vitamin deficiency. IV Plasma thiamine. Journal of Clinical Investigation 23, 297–302.

Carney M.W.P., Williams D.G. & Sheffield B.F. (1979) Thiamin and pyridoxine lack in newly admitted psychiatric patients. *British Journal of Psychiatry* **135**, 24–54.

Carr A.C., Wilson S.L., Ghosh A., Ancill R.J. & Woods R.T. (1982) Automated testing of geriatric patients using a microcomputer-based system. *International Journal of Man-Machine Studies* **17**, 297–300.

Chalmers F.W., Clayton M.M., Gates L.O., Tucker R.E., Wertz A.W., Young C.M. & Foster W.D. (1952) The dietary record — how many and which days? *Journal of American Dietetic Association* **28**, 711–17.

Chalmers T.C. (1975) Effects of Ascorbic Acid on the Common Cold: An evaluation of the evidence. *American Journal of Medicine* **58**, 532–6.

Chandra R.K. (1983) Nutrition, immunity and infection: Present knowledge and future directions. *Lancet* **1**, 688–91.

Chandra R.K. & Newberne P.M. (1977) *Nutrition, immunity and infection: Mechanisms of interactions.* Plenum Press, New York, London.

Chatamra K., Daniel P.M. & Lam D.K.C. (1985) Influx of ascorbic acid into the brain of the rat. *Journal of Physiology* **358**, 112p.

Chauhan M.S. & Dakshinamurti K. (1979) Fluorometric assay of pyridoxal and pyridoxal 5-phosphate. *Analytical Biochemistry* **96**, 426–32.

Chesney R.W., Mazees R.B., Hamstra A.J. & De Luca H.F. (1978) Reduction of serum 1, 25-dihydroxy-vitamin D in children receiving glucocorticoids. *Lancet* **2**, 1123–5.

Childs B. (1970) Sir Archibald Garrod's conception of chemical individuality: A modern appreciation. *New England Journal of Medicine* **282**, 71–7.

Childs B. & Der Kaloustian V.M. (1968) Genetic heterogeneity. *New England Journal of Medicine* **279**, 1205–12.

Chong Y.H. & Ho G.S. (1970) Erythrocyte transketolase activity. *American Journal of Clinical Nutrition* **23**, 261–6.

Clarke M., Clarke S., Odell A. & Jagger C. (1984) The elderly at home: Health and social status. *Health Trends* **16**, 3–7.

Cohen C. (1968) Zinc sulphate and bedsores. *British Medical Journal* **2**, 561.

Cohen E.L. & Wurtman R.J. (1976) Brain acetycholine, control by dietary choline. *Science* **191**, 561–2.

Cohen H. (1957) *Report of joint sub-committee on welfare foods.* HMSO, London.

Cole M.G. & Prchal J.F. (1984) Low serum vitamin B$_{12}$ in Alzheimer-type dementia. *Age and Ageing* **13**, 101–5.

Collins K.J., Exton-Smith A.N., James M.M. & Oliver D.J. (1980)

174   References

Functional changes in autonomic nervous responses with ageing. *Age and Ageing* **9**, 17–24.

Contractor S.F. & Shane B. (1968) Estimation of vitamin B6 compounds in human blood and urine. *Clinica Chimica Acta* **21**, 71–7.

Cook P.J., Exton-Smith A.N., Brocklehurst J.C. & Lempert-Barber S.M. (1982) Fractured femurs, falls and bone disorders. *Journal of Royal College of Physicians* **16**, 45–9.

Coon W.W. (1962) Ascorbic acid metabolism in postoperative patients. *Surgery, Gynaecology and Obstetrics* **114**, 522–34.

Corcino J.J., Waxman S. & Herbert V. (1970) Absorption and malabsorption of vitamin B_{12}. *American Journal of Medicine* **48**, 562–9.

Corless D., Beer M., Boucher D.J., Gupta S.P. & Cohn R.D. (1975) Vitamin D status in long stay geriatric patients. *Lancet* **1**, 1404–6.

Corless D., Gupta S.P., Switala S., Barragry J.M., Boucher B.J., Cohen R.D. & Diffey B.L. (1978) Response of plasma-25-hydroxyvitamin D to ultraviolet irradiation in long-stay geriatric patients. *Lancet* **2**, 649–51.

Cornford E.M., Braun L.D. & Oldendorf W.H. (1978) Carrier mediated blood-brain barrier transport of choline and certain choline analogues. *Journal of Neurochemistry* **30**, 299–308.

Cornford E.M. & Oldendorf W.H. (1975) Independent blood-brain barrier transport systems for nucleic acid precursors. *Biochimica Biophysica Acta* **394**, 211–19.

Corrigan J.J. & Marcus F.I. (1974) Coagulopathy associated with vitamin E ingestion. *Journal of American Medical Association* **230**, 1300–1.

Corwin L.M. & Schloss J. (1980) Influence of vitamin E on the mitogenic response of murine lymphoid cells. *Journal of Nutrition* **110**, 916–23.

Coughlan A.K. Hollows S.E. (1984) Use of memory tests in differentiating organic disorder from depression. *British Journal of Psychiatry* **145**, 383–6.

Crandon J.K., Lund C.C. & Dill O.B. (1940) Experimental human scurvy. *New England Journal of Medicine* **223**, 353–69.

Cremer J.E., Braun L.D. & Oldendorf W.H. (1976) Changes during development in transport processes of the blood-brain barrier. *Biochimica Biophysica Acta* **448**, 633–7.

Croker J.R. & Banyon G. (1981) Gastrointestinal bleeding — a major cause of iron deficiency in the elderly. *Age and Ageing* **10**, 40–3.

Curzon G., Friedel J. & Knott P.J. (1973) The effect of fatty acids on the binding of tryptophan to plasma protein. *Nature* **242**, 198–200.

Cusack B. & Denham M.J. (1984) Nutritional status and drug disposition in the elderly. In Roe D.A. (Ed.) *Drugs and nutrition in the geriatric patient*. 71–91. Churchill-Livingstone, Edinburgh.

Dalderup L.M. (1973) Ischaemic heart-disease and vitamin D. *Lancet* **2**, 92.

Daniel P.M., Love E.R., Moorhouse S.R. & Pratt O.E. (1977) The influence of age upon the influx of ketone bodies into the brain of the rat. *Journal of Physiology* **268**, 15–16.

Daniel P.M., Lam D.K.C. & Pratt O.E. (1981) Changes in the effectiveness of the blood-brain and spinal cord barriers in experimental allergic encephalomyelitis possible relevance to multiple sclerosis. *Journal of Neurological Sciences* **52**, 211–19.

Daniel P.M., Love E.R. & Pratt O.E. (1978) The effect of age upon the influx of glucose into the brain. *Journal of Physiology* **274**, 141–8.

Daniel P.M., Moorhouse S.R. & Pratt O.E. (1978) Post-natal changes in the transport of aromatic amino acids into the brain. *Journal of Physiology* **284**, 42–3p.

Darip M.D., Sirisinha S., Lamb A.J. (1979) Effect of vitamin A deficiency on susceptibility of rats to Angiostrongylus cantonensis. *Proceedings of Society for Experimental Biology and Medicine* **161**, 600–4.

Dastur D.K., Santhadevi N., Quadros E.V., Avari F.C.R., Wadia N.H., Desai M.N. & Barucha E.P. (1976) The B vitamins in malnutrition with alcoholism. A model of intervitamin relationships. *British Journal of Nutrition* **36**, 143–59.

Dattani J.T., Exton-Smith A.N. & Stephen J.M.L. (1984) Vitamin D status of the elderly in relation to age and exposure to sunlight. Human Nutrition: *Clinical Nutrition* **38C**, 131–7.

Davie M. & Lawson D.E.M. (1980) Assessment of plasma 25 hydroxy-vitamin D response to ultraviolet radiation over a controlled area in young and elderly subjects. *Clinical Science* **58**, 235–42.

Davies L. (1981) *Three score years and then.* Heinemann, London.

Davies L., Hastrop K & Bender A.E. (1973) Ascorbic acid in meals on wheels. *Modern Geriatrics* **3**, 390–4.

Davies P.E. & Mumford S.J. (1984) Cued recall and the nature of the memory disorder in dementia. *British Journal of Psychiatry* **144**, 383–6.

Deane B.R., Greenwood J., Lantos P.L. & Pratt O.E. (1984) The vasculature of experimental brain tumours. Part 4. The qualification of vascular permeability. *Journal of Neurological Science* **65**, 59–68.

Degvun M.S., Paterson C.R., Cohen C. & Johnson B.E. (1980) Possible value of fluorescent lighting in the prevention of vitamin D deficiency in the elderly. *Age and Ageing* **9**, 117–20.

Denson K.W. & Bowers E.F. (1961) The determination of ascorbic acid in white blood cells. A comparison of white blood cells, ascorbic acid and phenolic acid excretion in elderly patients. *Clinical Science* **21**, 157–62.

Dent C.E., Richens A., Rowe D.J.F. & Stamp T.C.B. (1970) Osteomalacia with long-term anti-convulsant therapy in epilepsy. *British Medical Journal* **4**, 69–72.

Department of Employment (1982) *Family Expenditure Survey 1981.* HMSO, London.

Department of Health and Social Security. (1970) Reports on Public Health and Medical Subjects No. 123. First report by the panel on nutrition of the elderly. HMSO, London.

Department of Health and Social Security. (1972) *A nutrition survey of the elderly. Reports on Medical Subjects No.* **3**. HMSO, London.

Department of Health and Social Security. (1978). *Prevention and Health: Eating for Health.* HMSO, London.

Department of Health and Social Security. (1979a). *Nutrition and Health in Old Age. Reports on Health and Social Subjects No.* **16**. HMSO, London.

Department of Health and Social Security. (1979b). *Recommended daily amounts of food energy and nutrients for groups of people in the United Kingdom. Reports on Health and Social Subjects No.* **15**. HMSO, London.

Department of Health and Social Security. (1980) *Report of Health and Social Subjects No. 19: Rickets and Osteomalacia.* HMSO, London.

Desai I.D. (1980) Assay methods. In Machlin L.J. (ed.) *Vitamin E, a comprehensive treatise.* 67–98. Marcel Dekker, New York.

De Wys W.D. & Walters K. (1975) Abnormalities of Taste Sensation in Cancer Patients. *Cancer* **36**, 1888–96.

Dibble J.B., Sheridan P., Hampshire R., Hardy G.J. & Losowsky M.S. (1982) Osteomalacia, vitamin D deficiency and cholestasis in chronic liver disease. *Quarterly Journal of Medicine New Series LI* **201**, 89–103.

Dickerson J.W.T. (1978) The interrelationships of nutrition and drugs. In Dickerson J.W.T. & Lee H.A. (eds) *Nutrition in the Clinical Management of Disease*, 308–31. Arnold, London.

Dickerson J.W.T. (1980) Interrelationships between diet and drugs. In Woods H.F. (ed.) *Topics in Therapeutics*, **6**, 127–36. Pitman Medical, Tunbridge Wells.

Dickerson J.W.T. (1981) Vitamin C and cancer. In Counsell J.N. & Horning D.H. (eds.) Vitamin C 349–58. Applied Science Publishers, London.

Dickerson J.W.T. (1983) Nutrition of the cancer patient. In Draper H. (ed.) *Advances in Nutritional Research*, **5**, 105– 31. Plenum, New York and London.

Dickerson J.W.T. (1984) Nutrition in the cancer patient: a review. *Journal of Royal Society of Medicine* **77**, 309–15.

Dickerson J.W.T. & Older M.J.W. (1982) The postoperative nutritional status of elderly orthopaedic patients with particular reference to vitamin A and zinc. *Proceedings of Nutritional Society* **41**, 122A.

Dobbelstein H., Korner W.R., Mempel W., Grosse-Wilde H. & Edel H.H. (1974) Vitamin B$_6$ deficiency in uraemia and its implications for the depression of immune response. *Kidney International* **5**, 233–9.

Dougados M., Zittoun J., Laplane D. & Castaigne P. (1983) Folate metabolism disorder in Kearns-Sayre syndrome. *Annals of Neurology* **13**, 687.

Dreizan S. (1979) Nutrition and the immune response — a review. *International Journal of Vitamin Nutrition Research* **49**, 220–0.

Drummond J.C. & Wilbraham A. (1958) The Englishman's Food. (Revised Hollingsworth D.). Cape, London.

Dreyfus P.M. (1962) Clinical application of blood transketolase determinations. *New England Journal of Medicine* **267**, 596–8.

Durnin J.V.G.A. & Womersley J. (1974) Body fat assessed from total body density and its estimation from skinfold thickness measurements on 481 men and women from 16–72 years. *British Journal of Nutrition* **32**, 77–79.

Dymock S.M. & Brocklehurst J.C. (1973) Clinical effects of water soluble vitamin supplementation in geriatric patients. *Age and Ageing* **2**, 172–6.

Eddy T.P. (1963) Nutritional values: Ascorbic Acid (Vitamin C) In *Food in Hospitals*. Oxford University Press, London.

Eddy T.P. (1972) A study of the relationship between Hess tests and leucocyte ascorbic acid in a clinical trial. *British Journal of Nutrition* **27**, 537–42.

Eddy T.P. & Taylor G.F. (1977) Sublingual varicosities and vitamin C in elderly vegetarians. *Age and Ageing* **6**, 6–12.

Edwin E.E. & Jackman R. (1973) Ruminal thiaminase and tissue thiamine in cerebrocortical necrosis. *Veterinary Record* **92**, 640–1.

Eickenberg H.U., Hahn H. & Opferkuch W. (1982) The influence of Antibiotics on the Host-Parasite Relationship. Springer-Verlag, Berlin.

Elwood P.C. & Bates J.F. (1972) Dentition and Nutrition. *Dental Practitioner* **22**, 472–9.

Elwood P.C. & Bird G. (1983) A photographic method of diet evaluation. *Human Nutrition: Applied Nutrition* **37A**, 474–7.

Elwood P.C., Burr M.L., Hole D., Harrison A, Morris T.K., Wilson C.I.D., Richardson R.W. & Shinton N.K. (1972) Nutritional state of elderly Asian and English subjects in Coventry. *Lancet* **1**, 1224–7.

Elwood P.C. & Hughes, D. (1970) Clinical trial of iron therapy on psychomotor performance in anaemic women. *British Medical Journal* **3**, 254–5.

Elwood P.C., Jacobs A., Pitman R.G. & Entwistle C.C. (1964) Epidemiology of the Paterson-Kelly syndrome. *Lancet* **2**, 716–20.

Elwood P.C., Shinton N.K., Wilson C.I.D., Sweetnam P. & Frazer A.C. (1971) Haemoglobin vitamin B_{12} and folate levels in the elderly. *British Journal of Haematology* **21**, 557–63.

Evans E. (1978) Quality of diet received by the patient. *Proceedings of Nutrition Society* **37**, 71–7.

Evans J.G. (1982) Epidemiology of proximal femoral fractures. *Recent advances in geriatric medicine*, Ch. 12, **2**, 201–14. Churchill-Livingstone, Edinburgh.

Evans R.M., Currie L. & Campbell A. (1980) Effects of platelets on apparent leucocyte ascorbic acid content. *Annals of Clinical Biochemistry* **17**, 252–5.

Evans R.M., Currie L. & Campbell A. (1982) The distribution of ascorbic acid between various cellular components of blood, in normal individuals, and its relation to the plasma concentration. *British Journal of Nutrition* **47**, 473–82.

Exton-Smith A.N. (1978) Nutrition in the elderly. In Dickerson J.W.T. & Lee A.H. (eds) *Nutrition and Clinical Management of Disease*, 73–104. Edward Arnold, London.

Exton-Smith A.N. & Stanton B.R. (1965) An investigation of the dietary of elderly women living alone. King Edward's Fund, London.

Fabris N., Pierpaoli W. & Sorkin E. (1972) Lymphocytes, hormones and ageing. *Nature* **240**, 557–9.

Faccini J.M., Exton-Smith A.N. & Boyde A. (1976) Disorders of bone and fracture of femoral neck. *Lancet* **1**, 1089–91.

Fenton-Lewis A. (1981) Fracture of neck of the femur: changing incidence. *British Medical Journal* **283**, 1217–20.

Ferris S.H., Sathananthan G. Reisberg B. & Gershon S. (1979) Long-term choline treatment of memory-impaired elderly patients. *Science* **205**, 1039–40.

Fisher B., Axelrod A.E., Fisher E.R., Lee S.H. & Calvanese N. (1958) The favourable effect of pyridoxine deficiency on skin homograft survival. *Surgery* **44**, 149–67.

Fioretto M. & Coward W.A. (1979) Pathogenesis of oedema in protein-energy malnutrition: the significance of plasma colloid osmotic pressure. *British Journal of Nutrition* **42**, 21–31.

Fox R.A. (1984) In Fox R.A. (ed.) Immunology and Infection in the Elderly, 289–309. Churchill Livingstone.

Fox R.H., Woodward P.M., Exton-Smith A.N., Green M.F., Donnison D.V. & Wicks M.H. (1973) Body temperature in the elderly: A national study of physiological, social and environmental conditions. *British Medical Journal* **1**, 200–6.

Fraser D.R. (1983) The physiological economy of vitamin D. *Lancet* 1, 969-72.

Fuerth J.H. (1971) Incidence of anaemia in full term infants seen in private practice. *Journal of Paediatrics* **79**, 560-2.

Funk C. (1912) The aetiology of deficiency diseases. *Journals of State Medicine* **20**, 341-68.

Furman K.I. (1972) Fluctuations in serum vitamin A. *Journal of Interdisciplinary Cycle Research* **3**, 217-23.

Gardner M.J. & Heady J.A. (1973) Some effects of within person variability. *Journal of Chronic Diseases* **26**, 781-95.

Garrod A. (1931) *Inborn factors in disease.* University Press, New York, Oxford.

Garry P.J., Goodwin J.S. & Hunt W.C. (1983) Iron status and anaemia in the elderly: new finding and a review of previous studies. *Journal of the American Geriatrics Society* **31**, 389-99.

Garry P.J., Goodwin J.S., Hunt W.L. & Gilbert B.A. (1982) Nutritional status in a healthy elderly population: Vitamin C. *American Journal of Clinical Nutrition* **36**, 332-9.

Girdwood R.H., Thomson A.D. & Williamson J. (1967) Folate status in the elderly. *British Medical Journal* **2**, 670-2.

Glatzle D., Korner W.F., Christeller S. & Wiss D. (1970) Method of the detection of a biochemical riboflavin deficiency by stimulation of $NADPH_2$-dependent glutathione reductase from human erythrocytes by FAD in vitro. *International Journal of Vitamin Nutrition Research* **40**, 166-83.

Glatzle D., Weber F. & Wiss O. (1968) Enzymatic test for the detection of riboflavin deficiency. NADPH-dependent glutathione reductase of red blood cells and its activation by FAD in vitro. *Experentia* **24**, 1122.

Glover J., Jay C. & White G.H. (1974) Distribution of retinol binding protein in tissues. *Vitamins and hormones* **32**, 215-35.

Goetzl E.J., Wasserman S.I., Gigli I & Austen K.F. (1974) Enhancement of random migration and chemotactic response of human leucocytes by ascorbic acid. *Journal of Clinical Investigation* **53**, 813-18.

Goldberg A. (1963) The anaemia of scurvy. *Quarterly Journal of Medicine* **32**, 51-64.

Goldberg E.M. & Connelly N. (1982) *The effectiveness of social care for the elderly.* Heinemann Medical, London.

Gopalan C. (1969) The Possible role for dietary Leucine in the pathogenesis of Pellagra. *Lancet* 1, 197-9.

Gosney M. & Tallis R. (1984) Prescription of contraindicated and interacting drugs in elderly patients admitted to hospital. *Lancet* 2, 564-7.

Greenwood J., Jeyasingham M., Pratt O.E., Ryle P., Shaw G.K. & Thomson A.D. (1984) Heterogeneity of human erythrocyte transketolase: a preliminary report. *Alcohol and Alcoholism* **19**, 123–9.

Greenwood J., Love E.R. & Pratt O.E. (1982) Kinetics of thiamine transport across the blood-brain barrier in the rat. *Journal of Physiology* **327**, 95–103.

Greenwood J. & Pratt O.E. (1983) Inhibition of thiamine transport across the blood-brain barrier in the rat by a chemical analogue of the vitamin. *Journal of Physiology* **336**. 479–86.

Greenwood J. & Pratt O.E. (1984) The effect of ethanol upon thiamine transport across the blood-brain barrier in the rat. *Journal of Physiology* **348**, 61p.

Griffiths L.L., Brocklehurst J.C., Scott D.L., Marks J. & Blackley J. (1967) Thiamine and ascorbic acid levels in the elderly. *Gerontologia clinica* **9**, 1–10.

Gross R.L. & Newberne P.M. (1980) Role of nutrition in immunological function. *Physiological Reviews* **60**, 188–302.

Gross R.L., Reid J.V.O., Newberne P.M., Burgess B., Marston R. & Hift W. (1975) Depressed cell-mediated immunity in megaloblastic anaemia due to folic acid deficiency. *American Journal of Clinical Nutrition* **28**, 225–32.

Gross S. (1976) Hemolytic anaemia in premature infants: Relationship to vitamin E, selenium, glutathione peroxidase and erythrocyte lipids. *Seminars in Hematology* **13**, 187–99.

Grzegorezyk P.B., Jones S.W. & Mistretta C.M. (1979) Age related differences in salt taste acuity. *Journal of Gerontology* **34**, 834–40.

Guggenheim K. & Buechler E. (1947) Nutritional deficiency and resistance to infection. *Hygiene* **54**, 103.

Hackett A.F., Yeung C.K. & Hill G.L. (1979) Eating patterns in patients recovering from major surgery — a study of voluntary food intake and energy balance. *British Journal of Surgery* **66**, 415–18.

Haddad J.G. & Chyu K.J. (1971) Competitive protein-binding radioassay for 25-hydroxycholecalciferol. *Journal of Clinical Endocrinology* **33**, 992–5.

Hahn T.J., Hendin B.A., Scharp C.R., Boisseau V.C. & Haddad J.G. (1975) Serum 25-hydroxycalciferol levels and bone mass in children on chronic anticonvulsant therapy. *New England Journal of Medicine* **292**, 550–4.

Hall J.C., Staniland J.R. & Giles G.R. (1980) Altered Taste Thresholds in gastrointestinal cancer. *Clinical Oncology* **6**, 137–42.

Hallbook T. & Lanner E. (1972) Serum-zinc and healing of venous leg ulcers. *Lancet* **2**, 780–2.

Hallbook T. & Hedelin H. (1977) Zinc metabolism and surgical trauma.

British Journal of Surgery **64**, 271–3.

Hamfelt A. (1964) Age variation of B_6 metabolism in man. *Clinica Chimica Acta* **10**, 48–54.

Hamilton P.D., Carey F.J. & Fitch C.D. (1977) Reduced inflammatory response with vitamin E deficiency. *Clinical Research* **25**, 618A.

Hankin J.J., Stallones R.A. & Messinger H.B. (1968) A short dietary method for epidemiologic studies III development of questionnaire. *American Journal of Epidemiology* **87**, 285–98.

Hanna S., Harrison M., MacIntyre I. & Fraser R. (1960) The syndrome of magnesium deficiency in man. *Lancet* **2**, 172–6.

Harman D., Heidrick M.L. & Eddy D.E. (1977) Free radical theory of ageing: effect of free-radical-reaction inhibitors on the immune response. *Journal of American Sociology* **25**, 400–7.

Harper C. (1979) Wernicke's encephalopathy: a more common disease than realised. A neuropathological study of 51 cases. *Journal of Neurology, Neurosurgery and Psychiatry* **42**, 226–31.

Harris A.B., Hartley J. & Moor A. (1973) Reduced ascorbic acid excretion and oral contraceptives. *Lancet* **2**, 201–2.

Hazell K. & Baloch K.H. (1970) Vitamin K deficiency in the elderly. *Gerontologia Clinica* **12**, 10–17.

Heaney R.P., Gallagher J.C., Johnston C.C., Neer R., Parfitt M. & Whedon G.D. (1982) Calcium nutrition and bone health in the elderly. *American Journal of Clinical Nutrition* **36**, 986–1013.

Heaton R.K., Baade L.E. & Johnson K.L. (1978) Neurological test results associated with psychiatric disorders. *Psychological Bulletin* **85**, 141–62.

Heinzerling R.H., Nockels C.F., Quarles C.L. & Tengerdy R.P. (1974) Protection of chicks against *E. coli* infection by dietary supplementation with vitamin E. *Proceedings of the Society for Experimental Biology and Medicine* **146**, 279–283.

Henzel J.H., de Woose M. & Lichti E.L. (1970) Zinc concentrations within wounds. *Archives of Surgery* **100**, 349–57.

Herbert V. (1967) Biochemical and hematologic lesions in folic acid deficiency. *American Journal of Clinical Nutrition* **20**, 562–9.

Herbert V. (1968) Nutritional requirement for vitamin B_{12} and folic acid. *American Journal of Clinical Nutrition* **21**, 743–56.

Hessov I. (1977) Energy and protein intake in elderly patients in an orthopaedic ward. *Acta Chirurgica Scandinavica* **143**, 145–9.

Heymsfield S.B., McManus C., Stevens V. & Smith J. (1982a) Muscle mass: reliable indicator of protein-energy malnutrition severity and outcome. *American Journal of Clinical Nutrition* **35**, 1192–9.

Heymsfield S.B., Stevens V., Noel R. & Smith J. (1982b) Biochemical composition of muscle in normal and semistarved human subjects:

relevance to anthropometric measurements. *American Journal of Clinical Nutrition* **36**, 131–42.

Hodges R.E. Baker E.M., Hood J., Sauberlich H.E. & March S.C. (1969) Experimental scurvy in man. *American Journal of Clinical Nutrition* **22**, 535–48.

Hodges R.E., Bean W.B., Ohlson M.A. & Bleiler R.E. (1962a) Factors affecting human antibody response. III. Immunological responses of men deficient in pantothenic acid. *Journal of Clinical Nutrition* **11**, 85.

Hodges R.E., Bean W.B., Ohlson M.A. & Bleiler R.L. (1962b) Factors affecting human antibody response. IV. Pyridoxine deficiency. *American Journal of Clinical Nutrition* **11**, 180.

Hodges R.E. & Canham J.E. (1971) Vitamin deficiencies; study of experimental vitamin C deficiency and experimental vitamin A deficiency in man. In Hansen R.G. & Munro H.N. (eds) *Problems of assessment and alleviation of malnutrition in the United States*. US Government Printing Office, Washington.

Hodges R.E., Hood J, Canham J.E., Sauborlich H F. & Baker E.M. (1971) Clinical manifestations of ascorbic acid deficiency in man. *American Journal of Clinical Nutrition* **24**, 432–43.

Hodgkin P., Kay G.H., Hine P.M., Lumb G.A. & Stanbury S.W. (1973) Vitamin D deficiency in Asians at home and in Britain. *Lancet* **2**, 167–72.

Hodkinson H.M. (1974) Osteomalacia and femoral fractures. *Lancet* **1**, 416.

Hodkinson H.M. & Exton-Smith A.N. (1976) Factors predicting mortality in the elderly in the community. *Age and Ageing* **5**, 110–15.

Hodkinson H.M., Stanton B.R., Round P. & Morgan C. (1973) Sunlight, vitamin D and osteomalacia in the elderly. *Lancet* **1**, 910–12.

Hoffbrand A.V., Newcombe B.F.A. & Mollin D.L. (1966) Method of assay of red cell folate activity and the value of the assay as a test for folate deficiency. *Journal of Clinical Pathology* **19**, 17–28.

Hoffman-Goetz L. & Kluger M.J. (1979) Protein deficiency: its effects on body temperature in health and disease status. *American Journal of Clinical Nutrition* **32**, 1423–7.

Hoffman-Goetz L., McFarlane D., Bistrian B.R. & Blackburn G.L. (1981) Febrile and plasma iron responses of rabbits injected with endogenous pyrogen from malnourished patients. *American Journal of Clinical Nutrition* **34**, 1109–16.

Holdsworth M.D., Dattani J.T., Davies L. & MacFarlane D. (1984) Factors contributing to vitamin D status near retirement ages. *Human Nutrition: Clinical Nutrition* **38C**, 139–49.

Hooper B., Whittingham S., Mathews J.D., Mackay I.R. & Curnow D.H.

(1972) Autoimmunity in a rural community. *Clinical and Experimental Immunology* **12**, 79–87.

Hopkins G. (1912) Feeding experiments illustrating the importance of accessory factors in normal dietaries. *Journal of Physiology* **44**, 425–60.

Horwitt M.K., Harvey C.C. & Dahm C.H. (1975) Relationship between levels of blood lipids, vitamins C, A and E, serum copper compounds and urinary excretions of tryptophan metabolites in women taking oral contraceptive therapy. *American Journal of Clinical Nutrition* **28**, 403–12.

Horwitt M.K., Harvey C.C., Dahm C.U. Jr. & Searey M.T. (1972) Relationship between tocopherol and serum lipid levels for the determination of nutritional adequacy. *Annals of New York Academy of Sciences* **203**, 223–36.

Howell N., Boldy D. & Smith B. (1979) Allocating the home help service. *Occasional papers in social administration No. 63*. Bedford Square Press, London.

Hughes D., Elwood P.C., Shinton N.K. & Wrighton R.J. (1970) Clinical trial of the effect of vitamin B_{12} in elderly subjects with low serum B_{12} levels. *British Medical Journal* **2**, 458–60.

Hughes R.E. (1980) Vitamin C. British Nutrition Foundation, London.

Hughes R.E. (1982) Recommended daily amounts and biochemical roles in the vitamin C, carnitine, fatigue relationship. In Counsell J.N. & Hornig D.H. (eds) *Vitamin C*, 75. Applied Science Publishers Ltd., London.

Hughes R.E., Hurley R.J. & Jones R.E. (1980) Dietary ascorbic acid and muscle carotene in guinea pigs. *British Journal of Nutrition* **43**, 385–8.

Hume E.M. & Krebs H.A. (1949) Vitamin A requirement of human adults: an experimental study of vitamin A deprivation in man. *United Kingdom Medical Research Council Special Report* **264**, London.

Hunt A. (1978) *The elderly at home*. OPCS. HMSO, London.

Hunt C., Chakravorty N.K. & Annan G. (1984) The clinical and biochemical effects of vitamin C supplementation in short-stay hospitalised geriatric patients. *International Journal of Vitamin Nutrition Research* **54**, 65–74.

Huque T. (1982) A survey of human liver reserves of retinol in London. *British Journal of Nutrition* **47**, 165–172.

Hurdle A.D.F. & Picton-Williams T.C. (1966) Folic acid deficiency in elderly patients admitted to hospital. *British Medical Journal* **2**, 202–5.

Hurwitz N. (1969) Predisposing factors in adverse reactions to drugs.

British Medical Journal **1**, 536–9.

Iber F.L., Blass J.P., Brin M. & Leery C.M. (1982) Thiamin in the elderly — relation to alcoholism and to neurological degenerative disease. American Journal of Clinical Nutrition **36**, 1067–82.

Ibrahim I.K. & Sutcliffe R.L.G. (1977) Diet and drugs may combine to produce hypomagnesaemia. Medical Geriatrics **7**, 6–12.

Inkovaara J., Gothoni G., Halttula R., Heikinheimo R. & Tokala O. (1983) Calcium, vitamin D and anabolic steroid treatment of aged bones: double-blind placebo-controlled long-term clinical trial. Age and Ageing **12**, 124–30.

Irvin T.T., Chattopadhyay D.K. & Smythe A. (1978) Ascorbic requirements in postoperative patients. Surgery, Gynaecology and Obstetrics **147**, 49–55.

Ivey S.P. (1982) Nutrition and cancer patients. Nursing **2**, 129–32.

Jacobs A. (1982) Non-haematological effects of iron deficiency. Clinical Haematology **11**, 353–64.

Jaeger R.G. & Muller O.M. (1963) Effect of malnutrition on susceptibility of rats to Trypanosoma cruzi. V. Vitamin A deficiency. Experimental Parasitology **14**, 9.

Jagerstad M., Norden A., Kvist K. & Westesson A.K. (1979) Vitamin B$_{12}$ Scandinavian Journal of Gastroenterology, Oslo, **14**, (suppl. 52), 191–5.

Jagerstad M. & Westesson E.K. (1979) Folate. Scandinavian Journal Gastroenterology, Oslo, **14**, (suppl. 52), 196–202.

James P.T., Bingham S.A. & Cole T.J. (1983) Epidemiological assessment of dietary intake. Nutrition and Cancer **2**, 203–11.

Jeliffe D.B. (1966) Assessment of the Nutritional Status of the Community. WHO Monograph Service No. **53**, Geneva.

Jenkins D.H.R., Roberts J.G., Webster D. & Williams E.O. (1973) Osteomalacia in elderly patients with fracture of the femoral neck. Journal of Bone and Joint Surgery **55B**, 575–80.

Jha G.J., Deo M.G. & Ramalingasurami I. (1967) Bone growth in protein deficiency. American Journal of Pathology **53**, 1111–21.

Johnson K.R., Jobber J. & Stonawski B.J. (1980) Prophylactic vitamin D in the elderly. Age and Ageing **9**, 121–7.

Jowsey J., Schenk R.L. & Reutter F.W. (1968) Some results of the effect of fluoride on bone tissue in osteoporosis. Journal of Clinical Endocrinology and Metabolism **28**, 869–74.

Jubiz W., Haussler M.R., McCain T.A. & Tomlan K.G. (1977) Plasma 1,25-dihydroxy-vitamin D levels in patients receiving anticonvulsant drugs. Journal of Clinical Endocrinology and Metabolism **44**, 617–21.

Junes P.G., Kauffman C.A., Bergman A.G., Hayes C.M., Kluger M.J. & Cannon J.G. (1984) Fever in the Elderly: Production of leukocyte pyrogen by monocytes from elderly patients. *Gerontology* **30**, 182-7.

Kallner A., Hartmann D. & Hornig D. (1979) Steady state turnover and body pool of ascorbic acid in man. *American Journal of Clinical Nutrition* **32**, 530-9.

Kaplan S.S. & Basford R.E. (1976) Effect of vitamin B_{12} and folic acid deficiencies on neutrophil function. *Blood* **47**, 805-8.

Kark J.D., Smith A.H., Switzer B.R. & Hanes C.G. (1981) Serum vitamin A (Retinol) and cancer incidence in Evans County, Georgia. *Journal of National Cancer Institute* **66**, 7-16.

Katakity M., Webb J.F. & Dickerson J.W.T. (1983) Some effects of a food supplement in elderly hospitalised patients. *Human Nutrition: Applied Nutrition* **37A**, 85-93.

Kataria M.S., Rao D.B. & Curtis R.C. (1965) Vitamin C levels in the elderly. *Gerontologia Clinica* **1**, 189-190.

Kato R. & Takanaka A. (1968) Effect of phenobarbital on electron transport system, oxidation and reduction of drugs in liver microsomes of rats of different age. *Journal of Biochemistry (Tokyo)* **63**, 406-8.

Kawasaki T., Miyata I & Nose Y. (1969) Thiamine uptake in *Escherichia coli*. II. The isolation and properties of a mutant of *Escherichia coli* defective in thiamine uptake. *Archives of Biochemistry and Biophysics.* **131**, 231-7.

Kay D.W.K., Beamish P. & Roth M. (1964) Old age mental disorders in Newcastle-upon-Tyne. *British Journal of Psychiatry* **110**, 146-58.

Kay D.W.K., Bergmann K., Foster E.M., McKechnie A.A. & Roth M. (1970) Mental illness and hospital usage in the elderly: a random sample followed up. *Comprehensive Psychiatry* **11**, 26-35

Keltz F.R., Kies C. & Fox H.M. (1978) Urinary ascorbic acid excretion in the human as affected by dietary fibre and zinc. *American Journal of Clinical Nutrition* **31**, 1167-71.

Kemm J.R. (1979) Meals on wheels and luncheon clubs. *Health Trends* **11**, 90-1.

Kemm J.R. (1981) Meals on wheels: when the face behind the food is needed more. *Health and Social Services Journal* **81**, 20-21.

Kemm J.R. & Allcock J. (1984) The distribution of supposed indicators of nutritional status in elderly patients. *Age and Ageing* **13**, 21-8.

Kemm J.R. Campbell G., Cotton R.E., Hosking D.J. & Boyd R.V. (1984) Osteoid in bones of elderly patients without bone disease. *Age and Ageing* **13**, 144-51.

Kershaw P.W. (1967) Blood thiamin and nicotinic acid levels in alcoholism and confusional states. British Journal of Psychiatry **113**, 387–93.

Kinsman R.A. & Hood J. (1971) Some behavioural effects of ascorbic acid deficiency. American Journal of Clinical Nutrition **24**, 455–62.

Kirk J.E. & Chieffi M. (1953a) Vitamin studies in middle-aged and told individuals. XI. The concentration of total ascorbic acid in whole blood. Journal of Gerontology **8**, 301–4.

Kirk J.E. & Chieffi M. (1953b) Vitamin studies in middle-aged and old individuals. XII. Hypovitaminemia C. Effect of ascorbic acid administration on the blood ascorbic acid concentration. Journal of Gerontology **8**, 305–11.

Klaui H. (1979) Inactivation of vitamins. Proceedings of Nutrition Society **38**, 135–41.

Klidjian A.M., Foster K.J., Kammerling R.M., Cooper A. & Karran S.V. (1980) Relation of anthropometric and dynamometric variables to serious postoperative complications. British Medical Journal **281**, 899–901.

Knox E.G. (1973) Ischaemic heart-disease mortality and dietary intake of calcium. Lancet **1**, 1465–67.

Krasner N. & Dymock I.W. (1910) Measurement of capillary resistance by a negative pressure technique and its relationship to buffy layer ascorbic acid levels. International Journal of Vitamin Research **40**, 427.

Krebs H.A. (1953) The Sheffield Experiment on the Vitamin C Requirement of Human Adults. Proceedings of the Nutrition Society **12**, 237–46.

Labadarios D., Obuwa G., Lucas E.G., Dickerson J.W.T. & Parke D.V. (1978) The effects of chronic drug administration on hepatic enzyme induction and folate metabolism. British Journal of Clinical Pharmacology **5**, 167–73.

Lancet Editorial (1980) Vitamin A and Cancer. Lancet **1**, 575–6.

Lancet Editorial (1980) Food poisoning in hospitals. Lancet **1**, 576–7.

Lancet Editorial (1980) Lecithin and memory. Lancet **1**, 293.

Landsberg L. & Young J.B. (1982) Effects of nutritional status on autonomic nervous system control. American Journal of Clinical Nutrition **35**, 1234–40.

Langar M.L. & Yearlich E. (1976) The effect of improved oral hygiene on taste perception and nutrition in the elderly. Journal of Gerontology **31**, 413–18.

Lanzkowsky P., Erlandson M.E. & Bezan A.I. (1969) Isolated defect of folic acid absorption associated with mental retardation and cerebral calcification. Blood **34**, 452–65.

References   187

Lawson D.E.M., Paul A.A., Black A.E., Cole T.J., Mandal A.R. & Davie M. (1979) Relative contributions of diet and sunlight to vitamin D state in the elderly. *British Medical Journal* **2**, 303–5.

Lawson D.H., Richmond A., Nixon D.W. & Rudman D. (1982) Metabolic Approach to Cancer Cachexia. *Annual Reviews of Nutrition* **2**, 277–301.

Layrisse M., Blumenfeld N., Dugarte I. & Roche M. (1959) Vitamin B_{12} and folic acid metabolism in hookworm infected patients. *Blood* **14**, 1269–78.

Lazarov J. (1977) Resorption of vitamin B_1. XII. Changes in the resorption and the phosphorylation of thiamine in rats in relation to age. *Experientia Gerontologica* **12**, 75–99.

Lee J., Kolonel L.N. & Hinds M.W. (1981) Relative merits of the weight-corrected for height indices. *American Journal of Clinical Nutrition* **34**, 2521–9.

Lehmann J. (1979) How to investigate tryptophan malabsorption and the value of repeated tryptophan loads. In Schou M. & Stromgren E. (eds) *Origin, Prevention and Treatment of Affective Disorders*. Academic Press, London.

Lehmann J., Persson S., Walinder J. & Wallin L. (1981) Tryptophan malabsorption in dementia. *Acta Psychiatrica Scandinavica* **64**, 123–131.

Leichter J., Angel J.F. & Lee M. (1978) Nutritional status of a selected group of free-living elderly people in Vancouver. *Canadian Medical Association Journal* **118**, 40–3.

Lennard T.W.J., Rich A.J., Wright P.D. & Johnston I.D.A. (1983) Cancer cachexia — a clinical entity? *Clinical Nutrition* **2**, 27–9.

Levander O.A. (1975) Selenium and chromium in human nutrition. *Journal of American Dietetic Association* **66**, 338–44.

Levi R.N. & Waxman S. (1975) Schizophenia, epilepsy, cancer, methionine and folate metabolism, Pathogenesis of schizophrenia. *Lancet* **2**, 11–13.

Lim H.L., Neale R.V. & Kemm J.R. (1984) Handling of vitamin C by elderly patients. *Proceedings of Nutrition Society* **43**, 78A.

Lind J. (1753) *A treatise on Scurvy*. Reprinted 1953. Edinburgh University Press.

Linden V. (1974) Vitamin D and myocardial infarction. *British Medical Journal* **3**, 647–50.

Lishman W.A. (1978) *Organic Psychiatry*. Blackwells, Oxford.

Lonergan M.E., Milne J.S., Maule M.M. & Williamson J. (1975) A dietary survey of older people in Edinburgh. *British Journal of Nutrition* **34**, 517–27.

Loh H.S. & Wilson C.W.M. (1971) The relationship between leucocyte ascorbic acid concentration and the total white blood cell count.

International Journal of Vitamin Nutrition Research **41**, 253.

Lopes J., Russell D.M., Whitwell J. & Jeejeebhoy N. (1982) Skeletal muscle function in malnutrition. American Journal of Clinical Nutrition **36**, 602–10.

Losowsky M.S., Walker B.E. & Kelleher J. (1974) Malabsorption in clinical practice. 67. Churchill-Livingstone, Edinburgh.

Lumeng L., Brashear R.E. & Li T.K. (1974) Pyridoxal 5-phosphate in plasma: source, transport and metabolic fate. Journal of Laboratory Clinical Medicine **89**, 334–43.

Lund B., Sorenson O.H. & Christensen A.B. (1975) 25-hydroxycholecalciferol and fractures of the proximal femur. Lancet **2**, 300–2.

Lundholm K., Holm G. & Schersten T. (1978) Insulin resistance in patients with cancer. Cancer Research **38**, 4665–70.

Lynch S.R., Berelowitz I., Seftel H.C., Miller G.B., Krawitz P., Charlton R.W. & Bothwell T.H. (1967) Osteoporosis in Johannesburg Bantu males: its relationship to siderosis and ascorbic acid deficiency. American Journal of Clinical Nutrition **20**, 799–807.

MacBurney M. & Wilmore D.W. (1981) Rational decision making in nutritional care. Surgical Clinics of North America **61**, 571–82.

McClung L.S. & Winter J.C. (1932) Effect of vitamin A-free diet on resistance to infections of Salmonella enteriditis. Journal of Infectious Diseases **51**, 475.

MacCuish A.C., Urbaniak S.J., Goldstone A.H. & Irvine W.J. (1974) PHA responsiveness and subpopulations of circulating lymphocytes in pernicious anaemia. Blood **44**, 849.

McEvoy A.W., Fenwick J.D., Boddy K. & James O.F.W. (1982) Vitamin B_{12} absorption does not decline with age in normal elderly humans. Age and Ageing **11**, 180–3.

MacGregor G., Smith S.J., Markanan N.D., Banks R.A. & Sagnella G.A. (1982) Moderate potassium supplementation in essential hypertension. Lancet **2**, 567–70.

McLaren D.S. (1980) Stores, Sumps and Sinks. Lancet **1**, 242–4.

MacLennan W.J. (1981) The problem of potassium. In Caird F.I. & Evans J.G. (eds). Advanced Geriatric Medicine **1**, 67–71. Pitman, London.

MacLennan W.J., Andrews G.R., MacLeod C. & Caird F.I. (1973) Anaemia in the elderly. Quarterly Journal of Medicine **42**, 1–14.

MacLennan W.J., Caird F.I. & MacLeod C.C. (1972) Diet and bone rarefaction in old age. Age and Ageing **1**, 131–41.

MacLennan W.J., Coombe N.B., Martin P. & Mason B.J. (1975a) The relationship of laboratory parameters to dietary intake in a long-stay hospital. Age and Ageing **4**, 189–94.

MacLennan W.J., Hall M.R.P. & Timothy J.I. (1980a) Postural hypotension in old age: is it a disorder of the nervous system or of blood vessels? *Age and Ageing* **9**, 25–32.

MacLennan W.J., Hall M.R.P., Timothy J.I. & Robinson M. (1980b) Is weakness in old age due to muscle wasting? *Age and Ageing* **9**, 188–192.

MacLennan W.J. & Hamilton J.C. (1977a) The effect of acute illness on leucocyte and plasma ascorbic acid levels. *British Journal of Nutrition* **38**, 217–23.

MacLennan W.J. & Hamilton J.C. (1977b) Vitamin D supplementation and 25-hydroxycholecalciferol concentrations in the elderly. *British Medical Journal* **2**, 859–61.

MacLennan W.J., Hamilton J.C. & Timothy J.I. (1979) 25-hydroxy vitamin D concentration in old people living at home. *Journal of Clinical and Experimental Gerontology* **1**, 201–15.

MacLennan W.J., Martin P. & Mason B.J. (1975b) Energy intake disability, disease and skinfold thickness in a long-stay hospital. *Gerontolgia Clinica* **17**, 173–80.

MacLennan W.J., Martin P. & Mason B.J. (1977) Protein intake and serum albumin levels in the elderly. *Gerontology* **23**, 360–7.

MacLennan W.J., Morris P. & Mopson B.J. (1975c) Causes for a reduced dietary intake in a long-stay hospital. *Age and Ageing* **4**, 175–80.

MacLennan W.J., Stevenson I.H. & Shepherd A.N. (1984) *Treatment in Clinical Medicine: The Elderly.* Springer-Verlag, New York.

MacLennan W.J., Timothy J. & Hall M.R.P. (1980) Vibration sense, proprioception and ankle reflexes in old age. *Journal of Clinical and Experimental Gerontology* **2**, 159–72.

McLeod R.D.M. (1972) Abnormal tongue appearances and vitamin status of the elderly — a double blind trial. *Age and Ageing* **1**, 99–102.

MacLeod C., Judge T.G. & Caird F.I. (1974) Nutrition of the elderly at home. ii. Intake of vitamins. *Age and Ageing* **3**, 209–14.

Maguire G.P. (1978) The psychological impact of cancer. In Downie P.A. (ed.) *Cancer Rehabilitation.* 172–8. Faber and Faber, London.

Manninger R. (1928) Zur bakteriologischen Differential-Diagnose zwischen Geflugelcholera und Huhnertyphus. *Deutsche Tierarztliche Wochenschrift* **36**, 870.

Manz H.J. & Robertson D.M. (1972) Vascular permeability to horseradish peroxidase in brain stem lesions of thiamine-deficient rats. *American Journal of Pathology* **66**, 565–576.

Manzoor M. & Runcie J. (1976) Folate-responsive neuropathy: report of 10 cases. *British Medical Journal* **1**, 1176–8.

Marsden C.D. (1978) The diagnosis of dementia. In Issacs B. & Port F. (eds) *Studies in Geriatric Psychiatry.* 99–118. John Wiley, Chichester.

Mason K.E. & Bergel M. (1955) Maintenance of Mycobacterium leprae in rats and hamsters fed diets low in vitamin E and high in unsaturated fats. *Federation Proceedings* **14**, 442.

Matkovic V., Kestial K., Simonovic I., Buzina R., Brodarec A. & Nordin B.E.C. (1979) Bone status and fracture rates in two regions of Yugoslavia. *American Journal of Clinical Nutrition* **32**, 540–9.

Maxwell J.D., Hodt P. & Taylor W.H. (1984) Portable chair for testing isometric muscle strength. *Lancet* **1**, 18–19.

Mayersohn M. (1972) Ascorbic acid absorption in man: Pharmaco kinetic implications. *European Journal of Pharmacology* **19**, 140–2.

Medical Research Council (1948) Vitamin C requirement of human adults. A preliminary report of the Vitamin C Subcommittee. *Lancet* **1**, 853–8.

Milne J.S., Lonergan M.E., Williamson J., Moore F.M.L., McMaster R. & Percy N. (1971) Leucocyte ascorbic acid levels and vitamin C intake in older people. *British Medical Journal* **4**, 383–6.

Mitchell C.O. & Lipschitz D.A. (1982) The effect of age and sex on the routinely used measurement to assess the nutritional status of hospitalised patients. *American Journal of Clinical Nutrition* **36**, 340–9.

Mitchell H.H. (1964) Adaptation to under-nutrition. *Journal of American Dietetic Association* **20**, 511–15.

Mobarhan S., Maiani G., Zanacchi E., Ferrino A.M., Scaccini C., Sette S. & Feroo-Luzzi A. (1982) Riboflavin status among rural children in Southern Italy. *Human Nutrition Clinical Nutrition* **36C**, 71–80.

Montgomery R.D., Haeney M.R., Ross I.N., Sammons H.G., Barford A.V., Balakrishnan S., Mayer P.P., Culank J.S., Field J. & Gosling P. (1978) The ageing gut: a study of intestinal absorption in relation to nutrition in the elderly. *Quarterly Journal of Medicine* **47**, 197–211.

Moore M.C., Judlin B.C. & Kennemur P. McA. (1967) Using graduated food models in taking dietary histories. *Journal of American Dietetic Association* **51**, 447–50.

Moore P.J., Margrall D. & Clark R.G. (1982) The significance of hypoalbuminaemia. In Wesdorp R.I.C. & Soeters P.B. (eds) *Clinical Nutrition 1981*, 227–232. Churchill-Livingstone, Edinburgh.

Morgan D.B. & Hullin R.P. (1982) The body composition of the elderly mentally ill. *Human Nutrition* **36C**, 439–49.

Mudd S.H. & Levy H.L. (1978) Disorders of trans-sulfuration. In Stanbury J.B., Wyngaarden J.B. & Frederickson D.S. (eds) *The Metabolic Basis of Inherited Disease*. 4th Edition. 458–503. McGraw-Hill, New York.

Muenter M. Perry H.O. & Ludwig J. (1917) Chronic Vitamin A Intoxication in Adults. *American Journal of Medicine* **50**, 129–36.

Munro H.N. (1981) Nutrition and Ageing. *British Medical Bulletin* **37**, 83-8.

Murphy F., Srivastava P.C., Varadi S. & Elwis A. (1969) Screening of psychiatric patients for hypovitaminosis B_{12}. *British Medical Journal* **3**, 559-60.

Nayal A.S., MacLennan W.J., Hamilton J.C., Rose P. & Kong M. (1978) 25-hydroxy vitamin D diet and sunlight exposure in patients admitted to a geriatric ward. *Gerontology* **24**, 117-22.

Nelson J.S. & Fischer V.W. (1982) Vitamin E. In Barker B.M. & Bender D.A. (eds). *Vitamins in Medicine*, Vol. **1**, 147-71. Heinemann, London.

Newberne P.M. & Gebhardt B.M. (1973) Pre- and Post-natal malnutrition and response to infection. *Nutrition Reports International* **7**, 407.

Newberne P.M., Hunt C.E. & Young V.R. (1968) The role of diet and the reticuloendothelial system in the response of rats to *Salmonella typhimurium* infection. *British Journal of Experimental Pathology* **49**, 448.

Newton H.M.V., Morgan D.B., Schorah C.V. & Hullins R.P. (1983) Relation between intake and plasma concentration of vitamin C in elderly women. *British Medical Journal* **287**, 1429.

Nichoalds E.E., Lawrence J.D. & Sauberlich H.E. (1974) Assessment of status of riboflavin nutrition by assay of erythrocyte glutathione reductase activity. *Clinical Chemistry* **20**, 624-8.

Nordin B.E.C. (1980) Calcium metabolism and bone. In Exton-Smith A.N. & Caird F.I. (eds) *Metabolic and Nutritional Disorders in the Elderly*. 123-45. John Wright, Bristol.

Nordstrom J.W. (1982) Trace mineral nutrition in the elderly. *American Journal of Clinical Nutrition* **36**, 788-95.

Offenbacher E.G. & Pi-Sunyer F.X. (1980) Beneficial effect of chromium-rich yeasts on glucose tolerance and blood lipids in elderly subjects. *Diabetes* **29**, 919-25.

Older M.J.W. & Dickerson J.W.T. (1982) Thiamine and the elderly orthopaedic patient. *Age and Ageing* **11**, 101-7.

Older M.J.W., Dickerson J.W.T. & Taylor J. (1981) The nutritional status of patients following surgical treatment for a femoral neck fracture. *Journal of Bone and Joint Surgery* **63B**, 641.

Older M.W.J., Edwards D. & Dickerson J.W.T. (1980) A nutrient survey in elderly women with femoral neck fractures. *British Journal of Surgery* **07**, 884-6.

Olson J.A. (1972) The biological role of vitamin A in maintaining epithelial tissues. *Israeli Journal of Medical Science* **8**, 1170-8.

OPCS (1973) (Office of Population Censuses and Surveys) *General*

Household Survey 1973. HMSO, London.

Panda B., Holmes G.F. & DeVolt H.M. (1964) Studies on coccidiosis in vitamin A nutrition of broilers. *Poultry Science* **43**, 154.

Papapoulos S.E., Clements T.L., Fraher L.J., Gleid J. & O'Riordan J.L.H. (1980) Metabolites of vitamin D in human vitamin D deficiency: effect of vitamin D_3 or 1, 25-dihydroxycholecalciferol. *Lancet* **2**, 612–15.

Parfitt A.M. (1983) Dietary risk factors for age related bone loss and fractures. *Lancet* **2**, 1181–4.

Parfitt A.M., Gallagher J.C., Heaney R.P., Johnston C.C., Neer R. & Whedon G.D. (1982) Vitamin D and bone health in the elderly. *American Journal of Clinical Nutrition* **36**, 1014–31.

Paterson C.R. (1980) Vitamin D poisoning. Survey of causes in 21 patients with hypercalcaemia. *Lancet* **1**, 1164–5.

Paterson C.R. & MacLennan W.J. (1984) Bone Disease in the Elderly. John Wiley & Sons, Chichester.

Pathy M.S., Pippen C.A.R. & Kirkman S. (1972) Free and intrinsic factor bound radioactive cyanobalmin. Simultaneous administration to assess the signifiance of low serum vitamin B_{12} levels. *Age and Ageing* **1**, 111–19.

Paul A.A. & Southgate D.A.T. (1979) In McCance and Widdowson (Eds) *Composition of Foods* HMSO, London.

Pauling L. (1970) Vitamin C and the common cold. San Francisco. W.H. Freeman.

Pearson W.N. (1967) Blood and urinary vitamin levels as potential indices of body stores. *American Journal of Clinical Nutrition* **20**, 514–25.

Pederson A.B. & Mosbech J. (1969) Morbidity of pernicious anaemia. *Acta Medica Scandinavica* **185**, 449–52.

Peto R., Doll R., Buckley J.D. & Sporn M.B. (1981) Can dietary beta carotene materially reduce human cancer rates? *Nature* **290**, 201–08.

Phair J.P. (1979) Ageing and Infection: a review. *Journal of Chronic Diseases* **32**, 535–40.

Phair J., Kauffman C.A., Bjornson A., Adams L. & Linnemann C.J. (1978) Failure to respond to influenza vaccine in the aged. Correlation with B cell number and function. *Journal of Laboratory and Clinical Medicine* **92**, 822–8.

Phillip G. & Smith J.F. (1973) Hypothermia and Wernicke's Encephalopathy. *Lancet* **2**, 122–4.

Piironen V., Varo P., Syvaoja E.L., Salminan K. & Koivistoinen P. (1983) HPLC determination of tocopherols and tocotrienols and its application to diets and plasma of Finnish men. *International Journal of*

Vitamin Nutrition Research **53**, 35-40.

Pincus J.H., Cooper J.R., Itokawa Y. & Gumbinus N. (1971) Subacute Necrotizing Encephalomyelopathy. Effects of thiamine and thiamine propyl disulphide. *Archives of Neurology* **24**, 511-17.

Pincus J.H., Solitaire G.B. & Cooper J.R. (1976) Thiamine triphosphate levels and histopathology. Correlation in Leigh disease. *Archives of Neurology* **33**, 759-63.

Plaitakis A., Hwang E.C., Van Woert M.H., Szilagyi P.I.A. & Berl S. (1982) Effect of thiamine deficiency on brain neurotransmitter substances. *Annals of New York Academy of Sciences* **378**, 367-80.

Platt B.S. (1963) Food in Hospitals. Oxford University Press.

Platt B.S., Eddy T.P. & Pellett P.L. (1963) Nutritional values: ascorbic acid (vitamin C). In *Food in Hospitals*, 69-73. Oxford University Press, London.

Poskitt E.M., Cole T. & Lawson D.E.M. (1979) Diet, sunlight and 25-hydroxyvitamin D in healthy children and adults. *British Medical Journal* **1**, 221-3.

Poulter J.M., White W.F. & Dickerson J.W.T. (1985) Ascorbic acid supplementation and five year survival rates in women with early breast cancer. *Acta Vitamiologica Enzymologica* **6**, 175-82.

Powell D.E.B., Thomas J.H. & Khan A.N. (1979) Assessment of chemical tests for faecal occult bleeding and correlation of results with presence or absence of anaemia. *Gerontology* **25**, 120-4.

Powers H.J. & Thurnham D.I. (1981) Riboflavin deficiencies in man: effects on haemoglobin and reduced glutathione in erythrocytes of different ages. *British Journal of Nutrition* **46**, 257-66.

Prasad J.S. (1980) Effect of vitamin E supplementation on leucocyte function. *American Journal of Clinical Nutrition* **33**, 606-8.

Pratt O.E. (1976) Transport of metabolizable substances into the living brain. In Levi B & Lajtha A. (eds) *Transport Phenomena in the Nervous System: Physiological and Pathological Aspects*. 55-75. Plenum Press, New York and London.

Pratt O.E. (1979) The kinetics of tryptophan transport across the blood-brain barrier. *Journal of Neural Transmission Supplement* **15**, 29-42.

Pratt O.E. (1980a) A new approach to the treatment of phenylketonuria. *Journal of Mental Deficiency Research* **24**, 203-17.

Pratt O.E. (1980b) The transport of nutrients into the brain: the effect of alcohol upon their supply and utilization. In Richter D. (ed.) *Addiction and Brain Damage*, 94-128.

Pratt O.E. (1981) The need of the brain for amino acids and how they are transported across the blood-brain barrier. In N.R. Belton & C. Toothill (eds). *Transport and Inherited Disease*, 87-122. MTP

Press, Lancaster, Boston, The Hague.

Pratt O.E. (1982) Transport inhibition in the pathology of phenylketonuria and other inherited metabolic diseases. *Journal of Inherited and Metabolic Diseases* 5, 75–81.

Prentice A.M. & Bates C.J. (1981) Biochemical evaluation of the E.G.R. test for riboflavin. 1) Rate and specificity of response in acute deficiency. *British Journal of Nutrition* 45, 37–52.

Pruzansky J. & Axelrod A.E. (1955) Antibody production to diphtheria toxoid in vitamin deficiency states. *Proceedings of Society for Experimental Biology and Medicine* 89, 323.

Puxty J.A.H. & Fox R.A. (1984a) In Fox R.A. (ed) *Immunology and Infection in the Elderly*. Fox R.A. Ed. 310–30. Churchill Livingstone.

Puxty J.A.H. & Fox R.A. (1984b) In Fox R.A. (ed.) *Immunology and Infection in the elderly*, p. 179–201. Churchill Livingstone.

Puxty J.A.H., Horan M.A. & Fox R.A. (1983) Necropsies in the Elderly. *Lancet* 1 1262–4.

Quick A.J. (1970) *Bleeding problems in clinical medicine*. W.B. Saunder & Co., Philadelphia.

Rajalakshmi R., Deodhar A.D. & Ramakrishnan C.V. (1965) Vitamin C secretion during lactation. *Acta paediatrica Scandinavica* 54, 375–382.

Raper C.G.L. & Chaudhury M. (1978) Early detection of folic acid deficiency in elderly patients. *Journal of Clinical Pathology* 31, 44–6.

Ray A.K. & Rao D.B. (1974) Calcium metabolism in elderly epileptic patients during anti-convulsant therapy. *Journal American Geriatric Society* 22, 222–5.

Read A.E., Gough K.R., Pardoe J.L. & Nicholas A. (1965) Nutritional studies on the entrants to an old people's home with particular reference to folic acid deficiency. *British Medical Journal* 2, 843–8.

Reggiani C., Patrini C. & Rindi G. (1984) Nervous tissue thiamine metabolism in vivo. I. Transport of thiamine and thiamine monophosphate from plasma to different brain regions of the rat. *Brain Research* 293, 319–29.

Royal College of Physicians (1984) Medication for the elderly. *Journal of the Royal College of Physicians of London* 18, 7–17.

Reynolds E.H. (1974) Iatrogenic nutritional effects on anticonvulsants. *Proceedings of Nutrition Society* 33, 225–9.

Reynolds E.H. (1976) Neurological aspects of folate and vitamin B_{12} metabolism. *Clinical Haematology* 5, 661–6.

Reynolds E.H. (1976) Folate and epilepsy. In Bradford H.F. & Marsden C.D. (eds) Biochemistry and Neurology, 247–52. Academic Press, London.

Reynolds E.H., Preese J. & Johnson A.L. (1971) Folate metabolism in epileptic and psychiatric patients. *Journal of Neurology, Neuro-surgery and Psychiatry* **34**, 726–32.

Rindi G., Patrini C., Comincioli V. & Reggiani C. (1980) Thiamine content and turnover rates of some rat nervous regions using labelled thiamine as a tracer. *Brain Research* **181**, 369–80.

Rindu G. & Ventura U. (1972) Thiamine intestinal transport. *Physiological Reviews* **52**, 821–7.

Robertson D.M. & Manz H.J. (1971) Effect of thiamine deficiency on the competence of the blood-brain barrier to albumin labelled with fluorescent dyes. *American Journal of Pathology* **63**, 393–9.

Robertson E.C. & Ross J.L. (1932) The effect of vitamin D in increasing resistance to infection. *Journal of Paediatrics* **1**, 69.

Roberts-Thompson I.C. Whittingham S., Youngchaiyud U. & Mackay I.R. (1974) Ageing, immune response and mortality. *Lancet* **2**, 368–70.

Robson L.C. & Schwarz M.R. (1975a) Vitamin B_6 deficiency and the lymphoid system. I. Effects on cellular immunity and *in vitro* incorporation of 3H-uridine by small lymphocytes. *Cellular Immunology* **16**, 135–44.

Robson L.C. & Schwarz M.R. (1975b) Vitamin B_6 deficiency and the lymphoid system. II. Effects of vitamin B_6 deficiency *in utero* on the immunological competence of the offspring. *Cellular Immunology* **16**, 145–52.

Rodriguez M.E. & Irwin M.I. (1972) A conspectus of research on vitamin A requirements of man. *Journal of Nutrition* **102**, 909–68.

Roe D.A. (1984) Adverse nutritional effects of OTC drug use in the elderly. In Roe D.A. (ed.) *Drugs and nutrition in the geriatric patient*, 121–133. Churchill-Livingstone, Edinburgh.

Roe F.J.C. (1981) Are nutritionists worried about the epidemic of tumours in laboratory animals? *Proceedings of Nutrition Society* **40**, 57–65.

Rose C.S. & Gyorgy P. (1952) Specificity of hemolytic reaction in vitamin E deficient erythrocytes. *American Journal of Physiology* **168**, 414–20.

Rosenberg I.H., Bowman B.B., Cooper R.A., Halsted C.H. & Lindenbaum J. (1982) Folate nutrition in the elderly. *American Journal of Clinical Nutrition* **36**, 1060–6.

Rosser M.N., Iversen L.I., Reynolds G.P., Mountjoy C.W. & Roth M. (1984) Neurochemical characteristics of early and late onset types of Alzheimer's disease. *British Medical Journal* **288**, 961–4.

Royal College of Physicians (1984) Medication for the elderly. *Journal of the Royal College of Physicians of London* **18**, 7–17.

Rushton C. (1978) Vitamin D hydroxylation in youth and old age. *Age and Ageing* **7**, 91–5.

Russell R.I. & Goldberg A. (1968) Effect of aspirin on the gastric mucosa of guinea pigs on a scorbutogenic diet. *Lancet* **2**, 606–8.

Sandstead H.H., Henriksen L.K., Gregor J.L., Prasad A.S. & Good R.A. (1982) Zinc nutriture in the elderly in relation to taste acuity, immune response and wound healing. *American Journal of Clinical Nutrition* **36**, 1046–59.

Sauberlich H.E., Dowdy R.P. & Skala J.H. (1974) *Laboratory tests for the assessment of nutritional status.* CRC Press, Florida.

Sauberlich H.E. (1975) Vitamin C status: Methods and findings. *Annals of New York Academy of Sciences* **258**, 438–50.

Schattenkerk M.E., Obertop H., Bruining H.A., van-Rooyen W. & van-Houten H. (1984) Early postoperative enteral feeding by a needle catheter jejunostomy after 100 oesophageal resections and reconstructions for cancer. *Clinical Nutrition* **3**, 47–9.

Schaumburg H., Kaplan J., Windebank A., Vick N., Rasmus S., Pleasure D. & Brown M.J. (1983) Sensory neuropathy from pyridoxine abuse: A new megavitamin syndrome. *New England Journal of Medicine* **309**. 445–8.

Schiffman S. & Pasternak M. (1979) Decreased discrimination of food odours in the elderly. *Journal of Gerontology* **34**, 73–9.

Schorah C.J., Morgan D.B. & Hullin R.P. (1983) Plasma vitamin C concentrations in patients in a psychiatric hospital. *Human Nutrition: Clinical Nutrition* **37C**, 447–52.

Schorah C.J., Newill A., Scott D.L. & Morgan D.B. (1979) Clinical effects of vitamin C in elderly patients with low blood vitamin C levels. *Lancet* **1**, 403–5.

Schorah C.J., Tormey W.P., Brooks G.H., Robertshaw A.M., Young G.A., Talukder R. & Kelly J.F. (1981) The effect of vitamin C supplements on body weight, serum proteins and general health of an elderly population. *American Journal of Clinical Nutrition* **34**, 871–6.

Schott G.D. & Wills M.R. (1976) Muscle weakness in osteomalacia. *Lancet* **1**, 626–629.

Schouten H., Statius Van Eps W. & Stuycker Boudier A.M. (1964) Transketolase in blood. *Clinica Chimica Acta.* **10**, 474–6.

Schrauzer G.N. & Rhead W.J. (1973) Ascorbic acid abuse: effects of long-term ingestion of excessive amounts on blood levels and urinary excretion. *International Journal of Vitamin and Nutrition Research* **43**, 201–11.

Scrimshaw N.S., Taylor C.E. & Gordon J.E. (1968) Interactions of nutrition and infection. *Monograph Series* **57**, World Health Organisation, Geneva.

Selby P.J., Chapman J.A.W., Etazadi-Amoli J., Dalley D. & Boyd N.F. (1984) The development of a method for assessing the quality of life of cancer patients. *British Journal of Cancer* **50**, 13–22.

Sen I. & Cooper J.R. (1976) The turnover of thiamine and its phosphate esters in rate organs. *Neurochemistry Research* **1**, 65–71.

Shaw D.M., MacSweeney D.A., Johnson A.L., O'Keefe R., Nadoo D., MacLeod D.M., Jog S., Preece J.M. & Crowley B. (1971) Folate and amine metabolites in senile dementia: a combined trial and biochemical study. *Psychological Medicine* **11**, 166–71.

Shaw D.M., Tidmarsh S.F., Sweene A.E., Williams S., Karajgi B.M., Elameer M. & Twining C. (1981) Pilot study of amino acids in senile dementia. *British Journal of Psychiatry* **139**, 580–2.

Sheltawy M., Newton H., Hay A., Morgan D.B. & Hullin R.P. (1984) The contribution of dietary vitamin D and sunlight to the plasma 25-hydroxyvitamin D in the elderly. *Human Nutrition: Clinical Nutrition* **38C**, 191–4.

Shilotri P.G. (1977a) Glycolytic, hexose monophosphate shunt and bactericidal activities of leucocytes in ascorbic acid deficient guinea pigs. *Journal of Nutrition* **107**. 1507–12.

Shilotri P.G. (1977b) Phagocytosis and leucocyte enzymes in ascorbic acid deficient guinea pigs. *Journal of Nutrition* **107**, 1513–17.

Shorvon S.D., Carney M.W.P., Chanarin I. & Reynolds E.H. (1980) The neuropsychiatry of megaloblastic anaemia. *British Medical Journal* **281**, 1036–8.

Sinclair H.M. (1982) Thiamin. In Barker B.M. & Bender D.A. (eds) *Vitamins in Medicine*, Vol. **2**. 114–62. Heinemann, London.

Smeets E.H.J., Muller H. & De Wael J. (1971) A NADH-dependent transketolase assay in erythrocyte hemolysates. *Clinica Chimica Acta* **33**, 379–86.

Smith F.R. & Goodman D.S. (1976) Vitamin A transport and human vitamin A toxicity. *New England Journal of Medicine* **294**, 805–8.

Smith F.R., Raz A. & Goodman D.S. (1970) Radioimmunoassay of human retinol-binding protein. *Journal of Clinical Investigation* **49**, 1754–61.

Smith W.B., Shobet S.B., Zagajeski E. & Lubin B.H. (1975) Alteration in human granulocyte function after in-vitro incubation with L-ascorbic acid. *Annals of New York Academic Sciences* **12**, 252–6.

Sneath P., Chanarin I., Hodkinson H.M., McPherson G.K. & Reynolds E.H. (1973) Folate status in a geriatric population and its relation to dementia. *Age and Ageing* **2**, 177–82.

Sorenson D.I., Devine M.M. & Rivers J.M. (1974) Catabolism and tissue levels of ascorbic acid following long-term massive doses in the guinea pig. *Journal of Nutrition* **104**, 1041–8.

Sorensen O.H., Lund B.I., Saltin B., Lund B.J., Andersen R.B., Hjorth L., Melsen F. & Mosckilde L. (1979) Myopathy in bone loss of ageing:

improvement by treatment with 1α-hydroxycholecalciferol and calcium. *Clinical Science* **56**, 157–61.

Soukop M. & Calman K.C. (1979) Nutritional support in patients with malignant disease. *Journal of Human Nutrition* **33**, 179–88.

Spector R. (1977) Vitamin homeostasis in the central nervous system. *New England Journal of Medicine* **296**, 1393–8.

Spector R. (1982) Thiamine homeostasis in the central nervous system. *Annals of New York Academy of Sciences* **378**, 344–53.

Sporn M.B. & Newton D.L. (1979) Chemoprevention of cancer with retinoids. *Federation Proceedings* **38**, 2528–34.

Srikantia S.G., Mohanram M. & Krishnaswamy K. (1970) Human requirements of ascorbic acid. *American Journal of Clinical Nutrition* **23**, 59–62.

Stamp T.C.B. & Round J.M. (1974) Seasonal changes in human plasma levels of 25–hydroxyvitamin D. *Nature* **247**, 563–65.

Stanton B.R. & Exton-Smith A.N. (1970) *A longitudinal study of the diet of elderly women.* King Edwards's Hospital Fund, London.

Stephens W.P., Klimiuk P.S., Warrington S. & Taylor J.L. (1982) Observations on the dietary practices of Asians in the United Kingdom. *Human Nutrition: Applied Nutrition* **36A**. 438–44.

Sterner R.T. & Price W.R. (1973) Restricted riboflavin: within subject behavioural effects in humans. *American Journal of Clinical Nutrition* **26**, 150–60.

Stock A.L. & Wheeler E.F. (1972) Evaluation of 2 meals cooked by large scale methods: a comparison of chemical analysis and calculation from food tables. *British Journal of Nutrition* **27**, 439–48.

Stokes P.L., Melikian V., Leeming R.L., Portman-Graham H., Blair J.A. & Cooke W.T. (1975) Folate metabolism in scurvy. *American Journal of Clinical Nutrition* **28**, 126–9.

Strachan R.W. & Henderson J.G. (1967) Dementia and folate deficiency. *Quarterly Journal of Medicine* **36**, 189–204.

Tattersall R.N. & Seville R. (1950) Senile purpura. *Quarterly Journal of Medicine* **19**, 151–9.

Taylor G.F. (1966) Diet of elderly women. *Lancet* **1**, 926.

Taylor G.F. (1968) A clinical survey of elderly people from a nutritional standpoint. In Exton-Smith A.N. Scott D.L. (eds) *Vitamins for the Elderly*, 51–6. John Wright, Bristol.

Taylor G.F., Eddy T.P. & Scott D.L. (1971) A survey of 216 elderly men and women in general practice. *Journal of Royal College of General Practitioners* **21**, 267–75.

Taylor T.V., Rimmer S., Day B., Butcher J. & Dymock I.W. (1974) Ascorbic acid supplementation in the treatment of pressure sores. *Lancet* **2**, 544–6.

Taylor W.H. (1972) Renal calculi and self-medication with multi-vitamin preparations containing vitamin D. *Clinical Science* **42**, 515–22.

Ten-state Nutrition Survey Reports, I-V, (1972) Centre for Disease Control Atlanta, Georgia, 30330.

Theologides A. (1979) Cancer cachexia. *Cancer* **43**, 2004–12.

Thomas D.E., Chung-A-On K.O., Dickerson J.W.T., Tidmarsh S.F. & Shaw D.M. Tryptophan and Nutritional Status of Patients with senile dementia. *Psychological Medicine*. In Press.

Thomson A.D. (1966) Thiamine absorption in old age. *Gerontologia Clinica* **8**, 354–61.

Thomson A.D. (1982) Alcohol-related structural brain changes. *Britain Medical Bulletin* **38**, 87–04.

Thomson A.D., Baker H. & Levy C.M. (1970) Patterns of 35S-thiamine hydrochloride absorption in the malnourished alcoholic patient. *Journal of Laboratory Clinical Medicine* **76**, 34–45.

Thomson A.D., Frank H. & Levy C.M. (1971) Thiamine propyl disulphide: absorption and utilization. *Annals of Internal Medicine* **74**, 529–34.

Threatt J., Nandy K. & Fritz R. (1971) Brain-reactive antibodies in serum of old mice demonstrated by immunofluorescence. *Journal of Gerontology* **26**, 316–23.

Thurnham D.I. (1972) Influence of glucose-6-phosphate dehydrogenase deficiency on the glutathione reduction test for ariboflavinosis. *Annals of Tropical Medicine and Parasitology* **66**, 505–7.

Thurnham D.I. (1981) Red cell enzyme tests of vitamin status: do marginal deficiencies have any physiological significance. *Proceedings of Nutrition Society* **40**, 155–63.

Thurnham D.I., Migasena P., Vudhivai N. & Supawan V. (1971) A longitudinal study of dietary and social influences on riboflavin status in pre-school children in northeast Thailand. *South East Asia Journal of Tropical Medicine and Public Health* **2**, 552–63.

Thurnham D.I. & Rathakette P. (1982) Incubation of NAD(P)H2: glutathione oxidoreductase (EC 1.6.4.2) with flavin adenine dinucleotide for maximal stimulation in the measurement of riboflavin status. *British Journal of Nutrition* **48**, 459–66.

Thurnham D.I., Rathakette P., Hambidge K.M., Munoz N. & Crespi M. (1982) Riboflavin, vitamin A and zinc status in Chinese subjects in a high risk area for oesophageal cancer in China. *Human Nutrition: Clinical Nutrition* **36C**, 337–49.

Tillotson J.A. & Baker E.M. (1972) An enzymatic measurement of the riboflavin status in man. *American Journal of Clinical Nutrition* **25**, 425–31.

Todd J.E. & Walker A.M. (1980) *Adult Dental Health Vol. I England and Wales 1968–1978*. HMSO, London.

200   *References*

Tomasi G.L. (1979) Reversibility of human myopathy caused by vitamin E deficiency. *Neurology* **29**, 1182–6.

Toothaker R.D. & Welling P.G. (1980) The effect of food on drug bioavailibility. *Annual Reviews of Pharmacology and Toxicology* **20**, 173–99.

Tredger J. (1982) Feeding the patient — a team effort. *Nursing* **4**, 92–3.

Truswell A.S. (1976) A comparative look at recommended nutrient intakes. *Proceedings of the Nutrition Society* **35**, 1–14.

Tyler H.A. (1984) *Studies on vitamin A and human cancer.* Ph.D. Thesis, University of Surrey.

Tyrell D.A., Craig I.W., Meade T.W. & White T. (1977) A trial of ascorbic acid in the treatment of the common cold. *British Journal of Preventive and Social Medicine* **31**, 189–191.

Vallance B.D., Hume R. & Weyers E. (1978) Reassessment of changes in leucocyte and serum ascorbic acid after acute myocardial infarction. *British Heart Journal* **40**, 64–8.

Vallance S. (1978) Leucocyte ascorbic acid and the leucocyte count. *British Journal of Nutrition* **41**, 409–11.

Vaughan J. (1975) *The Physiology of Bone.* Clarendon Press, Oxford.

Victor M., Adams R.D. & Collins G.H. (1971) *The Wernicke-Korsakoff syndrome.* Blackwell Scientific Publication, Oxford.

Vir S.G. & Love A.H.G. (1979) Nutritional status of institutionalised and non-institutionalised aged in Belfast, Northern Ireland. *American Journal of Clinical Nutrition* **32**, 1934–47.

Viswanathan C.T. & Welling P.G. (1984) Food effects on drug absorption in the elderly. In Roe D.A. (ed.) *Drugs and nutrition in the geriatric patient,* 47–116. Churchill-Livingstone, Edinburgh.

Vitale J. (1977) The impact of infection on vitamin metabolism: an unexplored area. *American Journal of Clinical Nutrition* **30**, 1473.

Vo-Khactu K.P., Clayburgh R.H. & Sandstead H.H. (1974) An improved NADH-dependent assay for assessing thiamine nutriture. *Journal of Laboratory Clinical Medicine* **83**, 983–9.

Wahl T.O., Gobuty A.H. & Lukert B.P. (1981) Long-term anticonvulsant therapy and intestinal calcium absorption. *Clinical Pharmacology Therapeutics* **30**, 506–12.

Wald N., Idle M., Boreham J. & Bailey A. (1980) Low serum vitamin A and subsequent risk of cancer. *Lancet* **2**, 813–15.

Walsh J.R., Cassel C.K. & Madler J.J. (1981) Iron deficiency in the elderly: it's often non-dietary. *Geriatrics* **36**, 121–32.

Walton J. (1982) *Essentials of Neurology,* 396–7. Pitman, London.

Wapnick A.A., Lynch S.R., Seftel H.C., Charlton R.W., Bothwell T.H. & Jowsey J. (1971) The effect of siderosis and ascorbic acid depletion on bone metabolism with special reference to osteoporosis in the

Bantu. *British Journal of Nutrition* **25**, 367–76.

Warnock L.G. (1976) The blood-brain barrier in thiamine deficiency. In Gubler C.J. *et al.* (eds) Thiamine 169–74. Wiley, New York.

Warnock L.G. & Burkhalter V.J. (1968) Evidence of malfunctioning blood-brain barrier in experimental thiamine deficiency in rats. *Journal of Nutrition* **94**, 256–68.

Waters W.E., Withey J.L., Kilpatrick G.S. & Wood P.H.N. (1971) Serum vitamin B_{12} concentrations in the general population: a ten-year follow-up. *British Journal of Haematology* **20**, 521–6.

Weather H.M. (1946) Resistance of cotton rats to the virus of poliomyelitis as affected by intake of vitamin A: Partial immunisation and sex. *Journal of Paediatrics* **28**, 14.

Weisman Y., Salama R., Harell A. & Edelstein S. (1978) Scrum 24, 25-dihydroxyvitamin D and 25-hydroxyvitamin D concentrations in femoral neck fractures. *British Medical Journal* **2**, 1196–7.

Welling P.G. & Tse F.L.S. (1982) The influence of food on the absorption of antimicrobial agents. *Journal of Antimicrobial Chemotherapy* **9**, 7–27.

Wells C.E.C. (1965) The clinical neurology of macrocytic anaemia. *Proceedings of the Royal Society of Medicine* **58**, 721–4.

Wells D.G. & Marks V. (1972) Anaemia and erythrocyte transketolase activity. *Acta. Haematology* **47**, 217–24.

Wertmann K., Crisley F.D. & Sarandria J.L. (1952) Complement-fixing murine typhus antibodies in vitamin deficiency states. III. Riboflavin and folic acid deficiencies. *Proceedings Society for Experimental Biology and Medicine* **80**, 404–6.

White F.R. (1945) Source of tumour proteins. II. Nitrogen balance studies of tumor-bearing mice fed a low nitrogen diet. *Journal of National Cancer Institute* **5**, 265–8.

Whitehead A. (1982) Measurement of change in the elderly. In Wheatley D. (ed.) Psychopharmacology of old age. Oxford Medical Publications 139–44.

Wigzell F.W., Alam A.K.M.S., MacLennan W.J. & Hamilton J.C. (1981) Osteomalacia and kyphosis. *Journal of Clinical and Experimental Gerontology* **3**, 166–73.

Willet W.C., Polk B.F., Underwood B.A., Stampfel M.J., Pressel S., Rosner B., Taylor J.O., Schneider K. & Hanes C.G. (1984) Relation of serum vitamins A and E and carotenoids to the risk of cancer. *New England Journal of Medicine* **310**, 430–4.

Willett W.C. & MacMahon B. (1984) Diet and Cancer an overview. *New England Journal of Medicine* **310**, 633–8 & 697–703.

Williams E.A.G., Cross R.L. & Newberne P.M. (1972) Amino acids and carbohydrate metabolism in Salmonella infection in dogs.

Federation Proceedings **31**, 657.

Williams R.S. & Hughes R.E. (1972) Dietary protein growth and retention of ascorbic acid in guinea pigs. *British Journal of Nutrition* **28**, 167–72.

Williams R.T. (1967) Comparative patterns of drug metabolism. *Federation Proceedings* **26**, 1029–39.

Williamson J. & Chaplin J.M. (1980) Adverse reactions to drugs in the elderly: a multicentre investigation. *Age and Ageing* **9**, 73–80.

Wilson T.S., Datta S.B., Murrell J.S. & Andrews C.T. (1973) Relation of vitamin C to mortality in a general hospital: a study of the effect of vitamin C administration. *Age and Ageing* **2**, 163–71.

Wilson T.S., Weeks M.M., Mukherjee S.K., Murrell J.S. & Andrews C.T. (1972) A study of vitamin C levels in the aged and subsequent mortality. *Gerontologia Clinica* **14**, 17–24.

Windsor A.C.W. & Williams C.B. (1970) Urinary hydroxyproline in the elderly with low leucocyte ascorbic acid levels. *British Medical Journal* **1**, 732–3.

Wissler R.W. (1947) The effects of protein depletion and subsequent immunisation upon the response of animals to pneumococcal infection. 1. Experiments with rabbits. *Journal of Infectious Diseases* **80**, 250.

Wood B., Breen K.S. & Pennington D.G. (1977) Thiamin status and alcoholism. *Australia and New Zealand Journal of Medicine* **7**, 475–84.

Wooton R., Brereton P.J., Clark M.B., Hesp R., Hodkinson H.M., Klenerman L., Reeve J., Slavin G. & Tellel-Yudilevich (1979) Fractured neck of femur in the elderly: an attempt to identify patients at risk. *Clinical Science* **57**, 93–101.

World Health Organisation (1967) Requirement of vitamin A, Thiamine, Riboflavine and Niacin. *Technical report series* **362**, World Health Organisation, Rome.

World Health Organisation (1972) Nutritional anaemias: report of a WHO group of experts. *Technical report series* **503**. World Health Organisation, Geneva.

Wright W.H. (1935) The relation of vitamin A deficiency to ascarisis in the dog. *Journal of Parasitology* **21**, 433.

Wu A., Chanarin I., Slavin G. & Levi A.J. (1975) Folate deficiency in the alcoholic — its relationship to clinical and haematological abnormalities, liver disease and folate stores. *British Journal of Haematology* **29**, 469–78.

Wynick D. & Bender D.A. (1981) The effect of oestrone sulphate on the activity of kynureninase *in vitro*. *Proceedings of Nutrition Society* **40**, 21A.

Yeung D.L. (1975) Relationship between cigarette smoking, oral contraceptives and plasma vitamins A, E, C and plasma triglycerides and cholesterol. *American Journal of Clinical Nutrition* **29**, 1216–21.

Yui Y., Itokawa Y. & Kawai C. (1980) Furosemide-induced thiamine deficiency. *Cardiovascular Research* **14**, 537–40.

Zweiman B., Schoenwetter W.F. & Hildeth E.A. (1966) The effect of the scorbutic state of tuberculin hypersensitivity in the guinea pig. I. Passive transfer of tuberculin hypersensitivity. *Journal of Immunology* **96**, 296–300.

Index